Pocke
ANA

GW01018135

PG Murphy, Editor

Southmead Hospital
Bristol, UK

SCIENCE PRESS

© Copyright 1994 Science Press Limited, 34–42 Cleveland Street, London, W1P 5FB, UK

British Library Cataloguing-in-Publication Data
A catalogue record for this book is available from the British Library

ISBN 1-85873-014-7

Project editor: Alison Taylor
Illustrator: Daniel Simmons
Typesetter: Tanya Mukerjee
Production: Rebecca Spencer
Printed in Spain by TALLERES GRAFICOS HOSTENCH S.A.

CONTENTS

ABBREVIATIONS LIST

ACh	acetylcholine
AChE	acetyl cholinesterase
ADH	antidiuretic hormone
AF	atrial fibrillation
ALT	alanine transaminase
APLT	activated partial thromboplastin time
ASA	American Society of Anesthesiology
AST	aspartate transaminase
AV	atrioventricular
BMI	body mass index
BSA	body surface area
CEPOD	Confidential Enquiry into Perioperative Deaths
CN^-	cyanide
CNS	central nervous system
CO	cardiac output
COAD	chronic obstructive airways disease
CPAP	continuous positive airway pressure
CPK	creatinine phosphokinase
CPR	cardiopulmonary resuscitation
CVP	central venous pressure
CVS	cardiovascular system
DA_1	dopamine$_1$ (receptor)
DDAVP	1-deamino-D-arginine vasopressin
DIC	disseminated intravascular coagulation
2,3–DPG	2,3-diphosphoglycerate
DVT	deep vein thrombosis
ECF	extracellular fluid
ECG	electrocardiogram
EMG	electromyogram
EMLA	eutectic mixture of lignocaine and prilocaine
ENT	ear, nose and throat

ETT	endotracheal tube
FBC	full blood count
FEV	forced expired volume
FFP	fresh frozen plasma
FRC	functional residual capacity
FVC	forced vital capacity
GA	general anaesthetic
GI	gastrointestinal
GIK	glucose insulin potassium (regimen)
HbF	foetal haemoglobin
HK	hexose kinase
HR	heart rate
IBW	ideal body weight
ICF	intracellular fluid
ICU	intensive care unit
im	intramuscular
IPPV	intermittent positive pressure ventilation
ITP	idiopathic thrombocytopenic purpura
iv	intravenous
LA	local anaesthetic
LAP	left atrial pressure
LV	left ventricle
LVEDP	left ventricular end diastolic pressure
LVSW	left ventricular stroke work
MAOI	monoamine oxidase inhibitors
MAP	mean arterial pressure
MH	malignant hyperthermia
MPAP	mean pulmonary artery pressure
MTX	methotrexate
NA	noradrenaline
NSAID	non-steroidal anti-inflammatory drugs
O/D	overdose

PAOP	pulmonary artery occlusion (wedge) pressure
pChE	pseudocholinesterase
PDEIII	phosphodiesterase III
PEEP	positive end-expiratory pressure
PEF	peak expiratory flow
PK	pyruvate kinase
PR	per rectum
PT	prothrombin time
PTR	prothrombin time ratio
RV	right ventricle
RVSW	right ventricular stroke work
SC	subcutaneous
SLE	systemic lupus erythematosis
SV	spontaneous ventilation
SVT	supraventricular tachycardia

TBW	total body weight
TIBC	total iron binding capacity
TT	thrombin time
U+E's	urea and electrolytes
URTI	upper respiratory tract infection
V_a	alveolar ventilation
VAE	venous air embolism
V_e	minute ventilation
VF	ventricular fibrillation
V_i	ventilatory index
V_{O_2}	oxygen consumption
V_t	tidal volume
VT	ventricular tachycardia
WPW	Wolff-Parkinson-White (syndrome)

NORMAL CARDIOVASCULAR PRESSURES

	Systolic (mmHg)	Diastolic (mmHg)	Mean
Peripheral venous	—	—	6–12
Right atrium	—	—	0–7
Right ventricle	14–30	0–7	12–17
Pulmonary artery	14–30	2–13	8–19
Pulmonary artery occlusion pressure	—	—	6–12
Left ventricle	100–150	2–12	—
Arterial	100–150	60–90	80–100

PAEDIATRIC CARDIOVASCULAR VALUES

	BP (mmHg)	Heart rate (bpm)	Hb (g/dl)	Blood volume (ml/kg)
Birth	80/60	140	18–20	65–105
Neonate	90/55	130	15–20	85
1 yr	95/65	120	9–13	80
2 yrs	95/65	110	9–13	80
7 yrs	105/65	100	13–14	80
14 yrs	120/70	85	Sex-related (= adult)	75

Cardiac index = 3–4 l/min/m^2
HbF 80% at birth, falling by 4% per week
P_{50} of HbF = 2.5 kPa
Sickledex test may give a false negative up to 6 mths

REGIONAL BLOOD FLOWS

	% Cardiac output	Blood flow (ml/min)	O_2 consumption (ml/100 g/min)
Brain	15	750	3.5
Heart	4	200	8
Kidneys	25	1250	6
Liver	30	1500	4
Skeletal muscle	20	1000	Variable
Rest	6	300	Variable
Total	100	5000	200–250 ml/min

OXYGEN TRANSPORT

The relationship between O_2 tension (PO_2) and O_2 saturation (SO_2) of the blood is described by the O_2Hb dissociation curve. Horizontal displacement of the curve results in an increase (left shift) or reduction (right shift) of affinity for O_2.

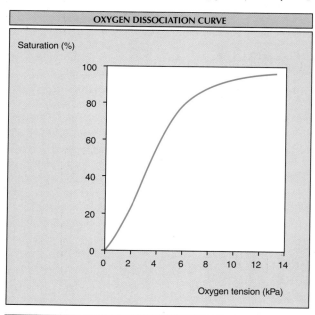

OXYGEN DISSOCIATION CURVE

Saturation (%)

Oxygen tension (kPa)

Left shift	Right shift	PO₂	SO₂
↓ PCO_2	↑ PCO_2	3.5	50
↓ temp	↑ temp	5.3	75
↓ [H^+]	↑ [H^+]	8.0	89
↓ 2,3–DPG	↑ 2,3–DPG	10.7	95
HbCO		13.3	98
HbF			

THE EFFECT OF TEMPERATURE, pH AND 2,3–DPG ON THE P_{50} VALUE

The position of the curve is described by the P_{50} value, the P_{O_2} at which HB is 50% saturated.

Temperature (°C)	40	37	34
P_{50} (kPa)	3.9	3.5	2.8
pH [(H^+) nmol/l]	7.7 (20)	7.4 (40)	7.2 (80)
P_{50} (kPa)	2.4	3.5	5.0
2,3–DPG	PK deficiency – high	anaemia	HK deficiency – low
P_{50} (kPa)	5.1	4.4	2.5

The O_2 content of blood, C_{O_2}, is dependent principally upon the Hb concentration and O_2 saturation of the blood:

$$C_{O_2} \text{ (ml/dl)} = \frac{\text{Hb (g/dl)}.SO_2 \text{ (\%)}.1.34}{100} + 0.023.P_{O_2} \text{ (kPa)}$$

Oxygen delivery to the tissues is determined by cardiac output (CO) and C_{O_2} thus:

$$D_{O_2} \text{ (ml/min)} = CO \text{ (l/min)}.10.C_{O_2}$$

OXYGEN CONSUMPTION

The body's oxygen consumption, V_{O_2}, can be measured using the following equation:

$$V_{O_2} \text{ (ml/min)} = CO \text{ (l/min)}.10.\frac{\text{Hb (g/dl)}.(S_aO_2 - S_vO_2).1.34}{100}$$

APPROXIMATE OXYGEN CONSUMPTIONS OF VARIOUS ORGANS

Organ	ml/min	% total	S_vO_2
Brain	46	18	65
Heart	23	9	23
Kidneys	18	7	90
Liver	66	26	72
Lungs	5	2	83
Muscle	64	25	62
Rest	33	13	48

PREDICTED LUNG FUNCTION VALUES

Forced vital capacity: Adult males (l)

Height			Age (yrs)					
cm	ft	in	20	30	40	50	60	70
160	5	3	4.17	4.06	3.84	3.62	3.40	3.18
168	5	6	4.53	4.42	4.20	3.98	3.76	3.54
175	5	9	4.95	4.84	4.62	4.40	4.18	3.96
183	6	0	5.37	5.26	5.04	4.82	4.60	4.38
191	6	3	5.73	5.62	5.40	5.18	4.96	4.74

Forced vital capacity: Adult females (l)

Height			Age (yrs)					
cm	ft	in	20	30	40	50	60	70
145	4	9	3.13	2.98	2.68	2.38	2.08	1.78
152	5	0	3.45	3.30	3.00	2.70	2.40	2.10
160	5	3	3.83	3.68	3.38	3.08	2.78	2.48
168	5	6	4.20	4.05	3.75	3.45	3.15	2.85
175	5	9	4.53	4.38	4.08	3.78	3.48	3.18

Forced expired volume at 1 sec: Adult males (l)

Height			Age (yrs)					
cm	ft	in	20	30	40	50	60	70
160	5	3	3.61	3.45	3.14	2.83	2.52	2.21
168	5	6	3.86	3.71	3.40	3.09	2.78	2.47
175	5	9	4.15	4.00	3.69	3.38	3.06	2.75
183	6	0	4.44	4.28	3.97	3.66	3.35	3.04
191	6	3	4.69	4.54	4.23	3.92	3.61	3.30

Forced expired volume at 1 sec: Adult females (l)

Height			Age (yrs)					
cm	ft	in	20	30	40	50	60	70
145	4	9	2.60	2.45	2.15	1.85	1.55	1.25
152	5	0	2.83	2.68	2.38	2.08	1.78	1.48
160	5	3	3.09	2.94	2.64	2.34	2.04	1.74
168	5	6	3.36	3.21	2.91	2.61	2.31	2.01
175	5	9	3.59	3.44	3.14	2.84	2.54	2.24

PREDICTED LUNG FUNCTION VALUES (cont.)								
Peak expiratory flow rates: Adult males (l/min)								
Height			**Age (yrs)**					
cm	ft	in	20	30	40	50	60	70
160	5	3	572	560	536	512	488	464
168	5	6	597	584	559	534	509	484
175	5	9	625	612	586	560	533	507
183	6	0	654	640	613	585	558	530
191	6	3	679	665	636	608	579	551
Peak expiratory flow rate: Adult females (l/min)								
Height			**Age (yrs)**					
cm	ft	in	20	30	40	50	60	70
145	4	9	377	366	345	324	303	282
152	5	0	403	392	371	350	329	308
160	5	3	433	422	401	380	359	338
168	5	6	459	448	427	406	385	364
175	5	9	489	478	457	436	415	394

FEV₁/FVC: normal > 75%
    restrictive lung disease > 60% (FVC reduced)
    obstructive lung disease < 50% (FVC near normal)

ACID-BASE BALANCE AND BLOOD GAS ANALYSIS

The pH scale of acidity was derived by chemists for chemists, encompasses an enormous range of $[H^+]$, and is not particularly suited to the description of biological acidity:

$$pH = - \log_{10} [H^+]$$

The range of $[H^+]$ compatible with life is 20–160 nmol/l; a pH change of 0.3 results in a doubling or halving of $[H^+]$ concentration.

pH	6.8	7.1	7.4	7.7
$[H^+]$ (nmol/l)	160	80	40	20

Renal control of $[HCO_3^-]$ and respiratory control of $[CO_2]$ combine to provide the body's most important buffering system, as described by the Henderson-Hasselbach equation:

$$pH = pK_a + \log\frac{[HCO_3^-]}{[CO_2]}$$

NORMAL ACID-BASE VALUES			
pH 7.36–7.44	H+ (nM) 43–36	P_aCO_2 4.6–6.0	metabolic status standard HCO_3^- 22–26 mM base excess ± 2.5 mM

APPROACH TO THE ANALYSIS OF ACID-BASE DISORDERS

Modern blood gas analysers measure pH, pCO_2 and pO_2. Estimates of metabolic status such as base excess and standard HCO_3^- are derived from these values of pH and P_aCO_2 using the assumption that the buffering activity of the body is acting normally. This activity may vary considerably in critically ill patients, due to changes in temperature and electrolyte concentrations, and it is therefore better to avoid over reliance on these potentialy misleading values and follow the scheme below:

1. define the acid-base disturbance from pH or [H+] measurement.
2. examine whether the change in P_aCO_2 is consistent or incompatible with this primary disturbance (i.e. is the disturbance primarily respiratory or metabolic in nature).
3. decide whether the primary change in pH has been compensated for by a secondary change in P_aCO_2 or HCO_3^- (using prediction formulae such as those presented in the table).

Plotting pH and P_aCO_2 on acid base diagrams such as the one below (which present 95% confidence limits for the *observed* relationship between pH and P_aCO_2 in a variety of acid-base disorders) may also aid analysis.

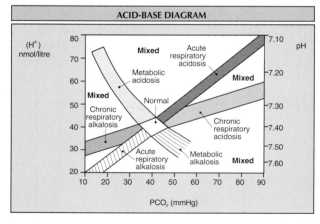

ACID-BASE DIAGRAM

BIOCHEMICAL FEATURES OF ACID-BASE DISTURBANCES

	Respiratory		Metabolic	
	Acidosis	**Alkalosis**	**Acidosis**	**Alkalosis**
1° disturbance	$\uparrow PCO_2$	$\downarrow PCO_2$	$\downarrow HCO_3^-$	$\uparrow HCO_3^-$
Acute response	$CO_2 + H_2O \rightarrow H^+ + HCO_3^-$		$H^+ + HCO_3^- \rightarrow CO_2 + H_2O$	
	$\uparrow HCO_3^-$: 1 mM/ 10 mmHg ΔPCO_2, $\uparrow H^+$: 0.8 x ΔPCO_2 nM, e.g. hypoventilation	$\downarrow HCO_3^-$: 2 mM/ 10 mmHg ΔPCO_2 $\downarrow H^+$: 0.8 x ΔPCO_2 nM, e.g. hyperventilation	$\uparrow PCO_2$; e.g. acidosis during controlled ventilation	$\uparrow PCO_2$ e.g. HCO_3^- administration during controlled ventilation
Chronic compensation	Renal: takes ≥ 48 hrs $\uparrow HCO_3^-$ 3–5mM/ 10 mmHg ΔPCO_2, $\uparrow H^+$: 0.3 x ΔPCO_2 nM, e.g. COAD	Renal: takes ≥ 48 hrs $\downarrow HCO_3^-$: 5 mM/ 10 mmHg ΔPCO_2, $\downarrow H^+$: 0.3 x ΔPCO_2 nM, e.g. long-term hyperventilation	Hyperventilation: $\Delta PCO_2 = 1$–1.3 x ΔHCO_3^- e.g. hyperventilating response to acute renal failure, diabetic ketoacidosis	Hypoventilation $\uparrow PCO_2 = 0.6$ x ΔHCO_3^- e.g. limited respiratory 'compensation' such as prolonged vomiting

PAEDIATRIC RESPIRATORY VARIABLES

Static variables
Static parameters generally equal adult values on a per kg basis.
Compliance is low because of the smaller number of alveoli; specific compliance
equals adult values.

tidal volume, V_t	70 ml/kg
V_d/V_t	0.3
FRC	30 ml/kg
lung compliance	5 ml/cmH$_2$O
specific compliance	0.55 ml/cmO$_2$/ml
airway resistance	
nose	19 cmH$_2$O/l/sec
mouth	7 cmH$_2$O/l/sec
closing volume	> FRC
Number of airways	14×10^6 (equals adult)
Number of alveoli	24×10^6 (much less than adult)

Dynamic variables
Dynamic parameters tend to be higher than adult values on a weight for weight
basis, reflecting the higher O_2 consumption.

minute ventilation, V_e	220 ml/kg/min
alveolar ventilation, V_a	140 ml/kg/min
ventilatory index, V_i	2.3 l/m^2/min
respiratory rate	20–60/min
oxygen consumption, VO_2	6–7 ml/kg/min
work of breathing	> adult

GASEOUS COMPOSITION OF RESPIRATORY GASES

kPa	Inspired air	Expired air	Alveolar air
PO$_2$	21.1	15.5	13.7
PCO$_2$	0.04	3.7	5.3
PN$_2$	79.5	75.7	76.0
PH$_2$O	0.7	6.3	6.3

GASEOUS COMPOSITION OF BLOOD		
kPa or ml/dl	**Arterial**	**Mixed venous**
PO_2	13.3	5.3
Co_2 total Hb-carried dissolved	20.0 19.7 0.3	15.0 14.9 0.1
PCO_2	5.3	6.0
C_{CO2} total carbamino HCO_3^- dissolved	50.0 2.5 45.0 2.5	55.0 3.7 47.4 2.9
PN_2	76.4	76.4
PH_2O	6.3	6.3

Alveolar gas equation:

$$P_aO_2 = P_IO_2 - \frac{P_aCO_2}{RQ}$$

(where RQ is the respiratory quotient)

Bohr equation for the estimation of alveolar dead space:

$$\frac{V_d}{V_t} = \frac{P_aCO_2 - P_eCO_2}{P_aCO_2}$$

Shunt equation:

$$\frac{Q_s}{Q_t} = \frac{C_cO_2 - C_aO_2}{C_cO_2 - C_vO_2}$$

(where C_cO_2 is estimated from P_aO_2)

Age-related changes in arterial oxygen tension

pre-operative:

$$104 - \frac{age}{4}\ mmHg$$

post-operative:

$$94 - \frac{age}{2}\ mmHg$$

9

COMPOSITION OF BLOOD PLASMA

Na^+	136–148 mmol/l	Total protein	62–82 g/l
K^+	3.6–5.0 mmol/l	Bilirubin	5–17 μmol/l
Cl^-	95–105 mmol/l	AST	8–40 IU/l
HCO_3^-	24–32 mmol/l	ALT	3–60 IU/l
Urea	2.5–6.6 mmol/l	Amylase	70–300 IU/l
Creatinine	62–124 μmol/l	Glucose	2.5–4.7 mmol/l
PO_4^-	0.8–1.1 mmol/l	Zn^{2+}	8–20 μmol/l
Ca^{2+}	2.12–2.61 mmol/l	CPK	50–100 IU/l
Mg^{2+}	0.7–1.0 mmol/l	Alkaline phosphatase	10–95 IU/l
Albumin	36–52 g/l	Osmolality	285–295 mosm/kg water
Globulin	24–37 g/l		

COMPOSITION OF BODY FLUIDS

Composition of body fluid compartments

Substance (mmol/l)	Intracellular fluid	Extracellular fluid	Substance (mmol/l)	Intracellular fluid	Extracellular fluid
Na^+	10	140	HCO_3^-	10	28
K^+	150	3.5	SO_4^{2-}	10	0.5
Ca^{2+}	Variable	2.3	PO_4^{3-}	40	1.2
Mg^{2+}	15	0.8	Protein	55	16
Cl^-	3	100	Anion gap	0	15

COMPOSITION OF VARIOUS BODY SECRETIONS

Fluid	Na^+ (mmol/l)	K+ (mmol/l)	Cl^- (mmol/l)	HCO_3^- (mmol/l)	Volume (l/day)	pH
Saliva	112	20	40	10–20	0.5–1.5	5–6.5
Gastric juice	50	15	140	0–15	2–3	1.5–3
Bile	145	5	100	40	0.5–1	6.5–8.5
Pancreatic juice	130	5	55	110	0.5–1	8
Ileal juice	140	10	80	20–40	1–3	6–7
Normal stools	30	60	30	20–60	0.1	6.5–8

COMPOSITION OF VARIOUS BODY SECRETIONS (cont.)

Fluid	Na$^+$ (mmol/l)	K$^+$ (mmol/l)	Cl$^-$ (mmol/l)	HCO$_3^-$ (mmol/l)	Volume (l/day)	pH
Diarrhoea	30–140	30–70	—	20–80	Variable	—
Sweat	10–50	10	10–40	—	0.5–1	—
Cerebrospinal fluid	140	4	130	25	0.2	7.32–7.40

BODY FLUID COMPARTMENTS (70 kg young adult male)

Compartment	% body weight	%TBW	Volume (l)	ml/kg
Extracellular fluid				
Plasma	4.5	7.5	3.2	45
Interstitial lymph	12.0	20.0	8.4	120
Dense connective tissue	4.5	7.5	3.2	45
Bone	4.5	7.5	3.2	45
Transcellular	1.5	2.5	1.0	15
Total	27.0	45.0	19.0	270
Intracellular fluid				
Erythrocytes	2.3	3.8	1.6	23
Total	33	55	23	330
Total body water	60	100	42	600

DISTRIBUTION OF BODY WATER: EFFECT OF AGE

Age (yrs unless otherwise stated)		% Total of body weight			
		Total body water	Extracellular fluid	Intracellular fluid	ECF/ICF
Premature neonate		80	—	—	—
Term neonate		75	42	33	1.27
1 month		70	32	38	0.84
1 yr		65	26	39	0.67
10 yrs		62	26	36	0.72
Males	25	60	27	33	0.82
	45	53	24	29	0.83
	65	54	26	28	0.93
	85	51	26	25	1.04
Females	25	51	23	28	0.82
	45	48	23	25	0.92
	65	44	22	22	1.00
	85	43	22	21	1.05

NORMAL ADULT HAEMATOLOGICAL VALUES

Haematocrit		White cell count	
Male	40–54%	Total	$4–11 \times 10^9$/l
Female	35–47%		
Haemoglobin		Neutrophils	$2.5–7.5 \times 10^9$/l
Male	13–18 g/dl	(40–75%)	
Female	11.5–16.5 g/dl		
Red cell count		Lymphocytes	$1.5–3.5 \times 10^9$/l
Male	$4.5–6.5 \times 10^{12}$/l	(20–45%)	
Female	$3.9–5.6 \times 10^{12}$/l		
Mean corpuscular volume	76–96 fl	Monocytes (2–10%)	$0.2–0.8 \times 10^9$/l
Mean corpuscular haemoglobin concentration	31–35 g/dl	Eosinophils (1–6%)	$0.04–0.44 \times 10^9$/l
Mean corpuscular haemoglobin	27–32 pg	Basophils (0–1%)	$0–0.1 \times 10^9$/l
Reticulocyte count	0.5–2% (of RBC)	Plasma viscosity	1.5–1.72
		Haemoglobin A_2	1.5–3.5%
Red cell diameter	6.7–7.7 μm	Haemoglobin F	< 2%
Red cell thickness	1.7–2.5 μm	Platelet count	$150–400 \times 10^9$/l

INVESTIGATIONS OF HAEMOSTASIS

Test	Normal range	Description
Platelet count	$150–450 \times 10^9$/l	
Bleeding time	3–9 mins	*In vivo* test of platelet activity
Prothrombin time (PT)	12–14 secs	Extrinsic pathway
Activated partial thromboplastin time (APTT)	35–45 secs	Intrinsic pathway
Thrombin time (TT)	10–12 secs	Common pathway
Reptilase test	17–19 secs	Heparin-independent assessment of common pathway
Euglobin clot lysis time	> 2 hrs	Tests presence of fibrinolytic activators in blood
Fibrinogen	2–4 g/l	
Fibrin(ogen) degradation products	< 10 mg/l	

INVESTIGATIONS OF HAEMOSTASIS (cont.)

Test	Description				
	PT	APTT	TT	Platelets	Reptilase test
Bone marrow failure, ITP, etc.	N	N	N	↓	N
Warfarin, vitamin K deficiency, liver disease, f_{VII} deficiency	↑	N/↑	N	N	N
$f_{VIII, IX}$ deficiency	N	↑	N	N	N
Massive transfusion	↑	↑	N	↓	N
Heparin treatment	↑	↑	↑	N	N
Disseminated intravascular coagulation (DIC), severe liver disease	↑	↑	↑	N/↓	↑

COAGULATION AND FIBRINOLYTIC SYSTEMS

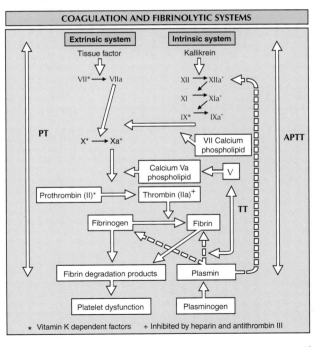

* Vitamin K dependent factors + Inhibited by heparin and antithrombin III

GUIDELINES FOR IDEAL BODY WEIGHT

Body Fat Content

Marathon runner	7%
Professional footballer	10%
Miss World	16%
Normal adult male	15–25%
Normal adult female	18–30%

Ideal Body Weight (IBW) (kg)
Adult males IBW = height (cm) – 100
Adult females IBW = height (cm) – 105
Body weight in children
Wt (kg) = 10 + 2 x age (yrs)

Body Mass Index (BMI)

BMI = Weight (kg)/height^2(m)

Normal	15–25
Obesity	27+
Morbid obesity	35+
Highest recorded	125

Obesity is diagnosed when weight is 120% of IBW. Morbid obesity is diagnosed when weight is > 200% of IBW, or when weight is IBW + 100 lbs/45.4 kg

RANGES OF NORMAL ADULT BODY WEIGHTS (kg)

Height (m)	Adult Males			Adult females		
	Average	Range	Obese	Average	Range	Obese
1.45	—	—	—	46.0	42–53	64
1.48	—	—	—	46.5	42–54	65
1.50	—	—	—	47.0	43–54	66
1.52	—	—	—	48.5	44–57	68
1.54	—	—	—	49.5	44–58	70
1.56	—	—	—	50.4	45–58	70
1.58	55.8	51–64	77	51.3	46–59	71
1.60	57.6	52–65	78	52.6	48–61	73
1.62	58.6	53–66	79	54.0	49–62	74
1.64	59.6	54–67	80	55.4	50–64	77
1.66	60.6	55–69	83	56.8	51–65	78
1.68	61.7	56–71	85	58.1	52–66	79
1.70	63.5	58–73	88	60.0	53–67	80
1.72	65.0	59–74	89	61.3	55–69	83
1.74	66.5	60–75	90	62.6	56–70	84
1.76	68.0	62–77	92	64.0	58–72	86
1.78	69.4	64–79	95	65.3	59–74	89
1.80	71.0	65–80	96	—	—	—
1.82	72.6	66–82	98	—	—	—
1.84	74.2	67–84	101	—	—	—
1.86	75.8	69–86	103	—	—	—
1.88	77.6	71–88	106	—	—	—
1.90	79.3	73–90	108	—	—	—
1.92	81.0	75–93	112	—	—	—

BODY SURFACE AREA

The body surface area (BSA) can be calculated by the Dubois and Dubois equation:

$$BSA = wt^{0.425} \times ht^{0.725} \times 0.007184$$

BSA = body surface area (m²) wt = weight (kg) ht = height (cm)

or by the Jacobson's equation, which is simpler and just as accurate:

$$BSA = (ht + wt - 60)/100$$

This information is most easily obtained clinically from nomograms relating height and weight.

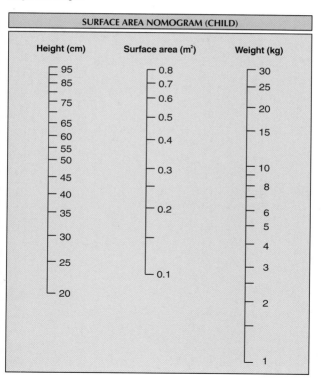

SURFACE AREA NOMOGRAM (CHILD)

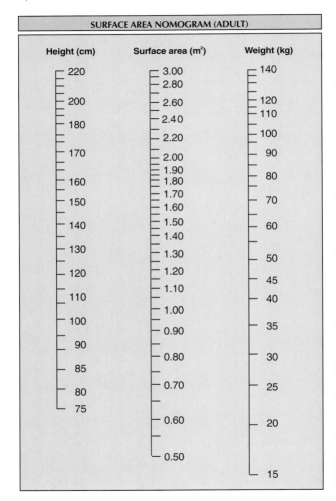

SURFACE AREA NOMOGRAM (ADULT)

Height (cm)	Surface area (m²)	Weight (kg)
220	3.00	140
200	2.80	120
180	2.60	110
170	2.40	100
160	2.20	90
150	2.00	80

WEIGHT CONVERSION TABLE

st	lb	kg	st	lb	kg	st	lb	kg
5	0	31.7	9	8	60.8	14	2	89.8
5	2	32.7	9	10	61.7	14	4	90.7
5	4	33.6	9	12	62.6	14	6	91.6
5	6	34.5	10	0	63.5	14	8	92.5
5	8	35.4	10	2	64.4	14	10	93.4
5	10	36.3	10	4	65.3	14	12	94.3
5	12	37.2	10	6	66.2	15	0	95.3
6	0	38.1	10	8	67.1	15	2	96.2
6	2	39.0	10	10	68.0	15	4	97.1
6	4	39.9	10	12	68.9	15	6	98.0
6	6	40.8	11	0	69.9	15	8	98.9
6	8	41.7	11	2	70.8	15	10	99.8
6	10	42.6	11	4	71.7	15	12	100.7
6	12	43.5	11	6	72.6	16	0	101.6
7	0	44.5	11	8	73.5	16	2	102.5
7	2	45.4	11	10	74.4	16	4	103.4
7	4	46.3	11	12	75.3	16	6	104.3
7	6	47.2	12	0	76.2	16	8	105.2
7	8	48.1	12	2	77.1	16	10	106.1
7	10	49.0	12	4	78.0	16	12	107.0
7	12	49.9	12	6	78.9	17	0	108.0
8	0	50.8	12	8	79.8	17	2	108.9
8	2	51.7	12	10	80.7	17	4	109.8
8	4	52.6	12	12	81.6	17	6	110.7
8	6	53.5	13	0	82.6	17	8	111.6
8	8	54.4	13	2	83.4	17	10	112.5
8	10	55.3	13	4	84.4	17	12	113.4
8	12	56.2	13	6	85.3	18	0	114.3
9	0	57.0	13	8	86.2	18	2	115.2
9	2	58.1	13	10	87.1	18	4	116.1
9	4	59.0	13	12	88.0	18	6	117.0
9	6	59.9	14	0	88.9	18	8	117.9

A pocket reference to anaesthesia

WEIGHT CONVERSION TABLE (cont.)

st	lb	kg	st	lb	kg	st	lb	kg
18	10	118.8	21	2	134.2	23	8	149.8
18	12	119.7	21	4	135.2	23	10	150.7
19	0	120.7	21	6	136.1	23	12	151.6
19	2	121.6	21	8	137.0	24	0	152.5
19	4	122.5	21	10	137.9	24	2	153.4
19	6	123.4	21	12	138.8	24	4	154.3
19	8	124.3	22	0	139.7	24	6	155.2
19	10	125.2	22	2	140.6	24	8	156.1
19	12	126.1	22	4	141.5	24	10	157.0
20	0	127.0	22	6	142.4	24	12	157.9
20	2	127.9	22	8	143.4	25	0	158.8
20	4	128.9	22	10	144.3	25	2	159.7
20	6	129.7	22	12	145.2	25	4	160.6
20	8	130.6	23	0	146.1	25	6	161.5
20	10	131.5	23	2	147.1	25	8	162.4
20	12	132.4	23	4	148.0	25	10	163.3
21	0	133.3	23	6	148.9	25	12	164.3

Weight: imperial – metric
1 kg = 2.20 lb   1 lb = 0.45 kg   1kg = 0.16 st   1st = 6.35 kg

1

HEIGHT CONVERSION TABLE

ft	in	m	ft	in	m	ft	in	m
2	6	0.76	4	0	1.22	5	6	1.68
2	7	0.79	4	1	1.25	5	7	1.70
2	8	0.81	4	2	1.27	5	8	1.73
2	9	0.84	4	3	1.30	5	9	1.75
2	10	0.86	4	4	1.32	5	10	1.78
2	11	0.89	4	5	1.35	5	11	1.80
3	0	0.91	4	6	1.37	6	0	1.83
3	1	0.94	4	7	1.40	6	1	1.85
3	2	0.97	4	8	1.42	6	2	1.88
3	3	0.99	4	9	1.45	6	3	1.91
3	4	1.02	4	10	1.47	6	4	1.93
3	5	1.04	4	11	1.50	6	5	1.96
3	6	1.07	5	0	1.52	6	6	1.98
3	7	1.09	5	1	1.55	6	7	2.01
3	8	1.12	5	2	1.58	6	8	2.03
3	9	1.14	5	3	1.60	6	9	2.06
3	10	1.17	5	4	1.63	6	10	2.08
3	11	1.19	5	5	1.65	6	11	2.11

Height: imperial – metric
1 inch = 2.54 cm   1 cm = 0.394 in   1 foot = 30.48 cm   1 m = 3.28 ft

DISTRIBUTION OF DERMATOMES

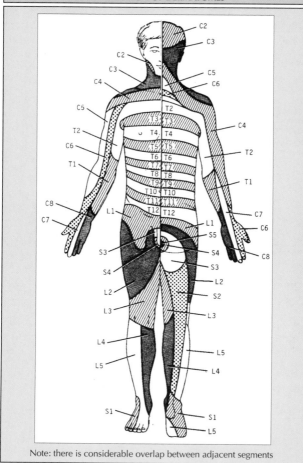

Note: there is considerable overlap between adjacent segments

VISCERAL INNERVATION				
Structure	Pathway	Sympathetic	Parasympathetic	Somatic
Thyroid	Cervical ganglia (mainly middle)	$C_{5,6}$		Overlying skin via cervical plexus C_{2-4}
Larynx	Cervical ganglia		Superior and recurrent laryngeal nerves	
Trachea, bronchi, lung parenchyma	Pulmonary plexus	T_{2-6}	Vagus	
Parietal pleura				Costal and peripheral diaphragmatic via intercostals T_{1-6}; central diaphragmatic and mediastinal via phrenic C_{3-5}
Heart	Middle and inferior cervical ganglia	T_{1-5}	Vagus	
Thoracic aorta	Cardiac and pulmonary plexuses	T_{1-6}	Vagus	
Oesophagus	Cervical ganglia, oesophageal and coeliac plexuses	T_{1-6}	Vagus	
Abdominal aorta	Coeliac plexus	T_6-L_2	Vagus	
Stomach		T_{6-9}		
Small intestine		$T_{9,10}$		
Pancreas		T_{6-10}		
Liver/ gallbladder		T_{6-9}		
Suprarenal glands		$T_{10}-L_1$		

VISCERAL INNERVATION (cont.)				
Structure	**Pathway**	**Sympathetic**	**Parasympathetic**	**Somatic**
Appendix, ascending and proximal two-thirds of transverse colon	Superior mesenteric plexus	T_{11}–L_1	Vagus	
Distal third of transverse colon, sigmoid colon and rectum	Inferior mesenteric plexus	$L_{1,2}$	Nervi erigentes. S_{2-4}	
Parietal peritoneum				Phrenic nerve, C_{3-5}; lower intercostals, T_{6-12}
Visceral peritoneum	From underlying viscera			
Kidneys Ureters	Coeliac and inferior mesenteric plexuses	T_{10}–L_1 T_{11}–L_2	Vagus	
Urinary bladder	Inferior hypogastric and vesical plexus	T_{11}–L_2		External sphincter via pudendal nerve S_{2-4}
Testes, epididymis, vas deferens	Renal, aortic and hypogastric plexuses	$T_{10,11}$		
Prostate/ prostatic urethra	Inferior hypogastric plexus	T_{11}–L_1	Nervi erigentes, S_{2-4}	
Ovaries	Renal, aortic and hypogastric plexuses	$T_{10,11}$		
Fallopian tubes Uterus	Ovarian and hypogastric plexuses	T_{10}–L_1 T_{11}–L_1		
Vagina	Inferior hypogastric and utero vaginal plexuses	$L_{1,2}$		Pudendal nerve, S_{2-4}

HAEMATOLOGICAL AND BIOCHEMICAL CHANGES DURING PREGNANCY

Haematology	Non-pregnant	Weeks of pregnancy		
		20	30	40
Blood volume (l)	4.0	4.6	5.5	5.7
Erythrocyte volume (l)	1.4	1.5	1.65	1.8
Red blood cells (10^{12}/l)	4.5	4.0	3.7	4.0
White blood cells (10^9/l)	7.2	9.4	10.7	10.4
Haemoglobin (g/dl)	13.5	12.0	11.5	12.0
Serum Fe^{2+} (mg/l)	1.2	1.0	0.9	0.9
Serum folate (µg/l)	10.0	7.0	6.0	6.0
Total iron binding capacity (TIBC) (µmol/l)	50.0	40.0	60.0	70.0
Biochemistry				
Na^+ (mmol/l)	138.0	136.0	137.0	136.0
K^+ (mmol/l)	4.3	4.0	4.1	4.2
Ca^{2+} (mmol/l)	2.5	2.5	2.28	2.30
Colloid osmotic pressure (cmH$_2$O)	37.0	32.0	31.0	31.0
Albumin (g/l)	35.0	28.0	26.0	25.0
Total protein (g/l)	70.0	60.0	61.0	62.0
Osmolality (mosmol/kg water)	281.0	283.0	280.0	280.0
Liver function tests				
Total bilirubin (µmol/l)	4–16	0.5–16	0.5–16	0.5–16
Alkaline phosphatase (IU/l)	16–24	16–44	16–60	20–100

A pocket reference to anaesthesia

VOLATILE ANAESTHETIC AGENTS

	Nitrous oxide	Enflurane	Isoflurane	Halothane	Sevoflurane	Desflurane
Formula	N_2O	CHF_2OCF_2CHFCl	$CHF_2OCHClCF_3$	$CF_3CHBrCl$	$CH_2FOCH(CF_3)_2$	$CHF_2OCHFCF_3$
Molecular weight	44.0	184.5	184.5	197.4	200.1	168.0
Specific volume	–	200	228	200	–	–
Boiling point (°C)	–88.5	56.5	48.5	50.2	58.5	23.5
Saturated vapour pressure at 20°C (kPa)	5200	22.9	31.9	32.5	21.3	88.5
Partition coefficients						
Blood/gas (37°C)	0.5	1.9	1.4	2.3	0.6	0.4
Brain/gas (37°C)	1.1	2.6	2.1	4.8	1.1	0.5
Olive oil/gas (37°C)	1.93	96.0	91.0	224	53.4	18.7
Lecithin/gas (37°C)	–	47.9	56.7	98.6	27.3	13.4
MAC in 100% O_2	NA	1.68	1.15	0.76	2.00	6–7.25
MAC in 66% N_2O	NA	0.57	0.56	0.29	0.66	2.8–4
Preservative	None	None	None	Thymol	None	None
Stability in soda lime	Stable	Stable	Stable	?Stable	?Unstable	Stable
% recovered as metabolite	Stable	2.4	0.2	> 20	2.0	0.02

INTRAVENOUS ANAESTHESIA

Various regimens describe maintenance of anaesthesia using continuous infusions of propofol in both ventilated and spontaneously breathing patients

Surgery	Induction (mg/kg)	Maintenance (mg/kg/hr)	Analgesia	Ventilated
ENT. head and neck[1]	2–2.5	12 → 9 → 6 at 10 min intervals	alfentanil, fentanyl	Yes
Body surface[2]	1	10 → 8 → 6 at 10 min intervals	N₂O + fentanyl	Yes
Body surface[3]	2.5	12 → 9 then titrated to response	N₂O	No
Minor urological[4]	1–2	10 → 5 after 10 mins	N₂O + NSAI	No

During prolonged procedures the maintenance dose may be reduced down to 4 mg/kg/hr according to clinical response. Doses of 1–4 mg/kg/hr may be used to provide sedation

Alfentanil may also be delivered in infusion: bolus = 50 mg/kg; infusion = 50 mg/kg/hr

References
1. De Grood, et al. Anaesthesia 1987, 42:366–372
   Ledderose, et al. Anaesthesia 1988, 43 (suppl):89–91.
   Gold, et al. J Clin Anaesth 1989, 1:272–276.
2. Roberts, et al. Anaesthesia 1988, 43 (suppl):14–17.
3. Sear, et al. Anaesthesia 1988, 43 (suppl):18–22.
4. Murphy PG. Unpublished data.

PAEDIATRIC DRUGS

Premedication

EMLA* cream and the unrestricted access of parents to the anaesthetic room have considerably reduced the need for sedative premedication, although it may still be useful in children making repeated visits to theatre. In addition, many practitioners have abandoned the routine use of anticholinergic drugs, arguing that they obtund a useful physiological indication of hypoxia; they should also be used with caution if the child is tachycardic or pyrexial.

atropine: 20 µg/kg im 45 mins pre-operatively
50 µg/kg orally, 2 hrs pre-operatively
or according to the following scheme

Weight	Dose (µg) im
< 2.5	150
2.5–10	200
10–15	300
15–20	400
> 20	500

* eutectic mixture of lignocaine and prilocaine; apply 60 mins before venepuncture

PAEDIATRIC DRUGS (cont.)

Sedative premedication

diazepam	0.1 mg/kg, orally 90 mins pre-operatively
triclofos	50–100 mg/kg, orally 2 hrs pre-operatively to maximum of 1 g
trimeprazine	2–4 mg/kg, orally 2 hrs pre-operatively
temazepam	0.3–0.5 mg/kg, orally 60–90 mins pre-operatively

Induction agents

propofol	2–5 mg/kg	methohexitone	1–1.5 mg/kg
thiopentone	4–8 mg/kg	ketamine	2 mg/kg iv
etomidate	0.3 mg/kg		10 mg/kg im/orally/pr

Muscle relaxants

Depolarising:

suxamethonium	1–2 mg/kg iv
	10 mg/kg im (particularly intraglossal)

Non-depolarising (reduce dose in neonates):

atracurium	0.5 mg/kg bolus	0.5 mg/kg/hr infusion
vecuronium	0.1 mg/kg bolus	0.1 mg/kg/hr
mivacurium	0.1–0.2 mg/kg bolus	0.6–1.0 mg/kg/hr
pancuronium	0.1 mg/kg	
curare	0.5 mg/kg	

Intra-operative analgesia

codeine	1 mg/kg im (not iv)	morphine	0.1–0.2 mg/kg
fentanyl	1–3 µg/kg	pethidine	1 mg/kg

Caudal regional analgesia

Sacral	0.5 ml/kg 0.25% bupivacaine
Lumbar	1 ml/kg 0.25% bupivacaine
T_{10}	1.25 ml/kg 0.25% bupivacaine

Reversal of muscle relaxants

neostigmine	50 µg/kg
atropine	20 µg/kg
glycopyrollate	10 µg/kg

e.g. make up 2.5 mg neostigmine with 500 µg glycopyrollate or 1.2 mg atropine to 10 ml; give 1 ml of the mixture for each 5 kg body weight.

PAEDIATRIC DRUGS (cont.)

Opioid antagonists

naloxone	1.5–3 μg/kg iv	
newborn	10 μg < 2 kg im	20 μg > 2 kg im

Anti-emetics

droperidol   25–50 μg/kg (20 μg/kg for day case surgery)
metoclopramide 0.5 mg/kg in three divided doses, im/iv/orally

Post-operative analgesia

paracetamol   10–15 mg/kg 4 hrly (max 4 doses/day)
'Calpol' = 120 mg/5ml
6 mths–1 yr   2.5–5 ml
1–6 yrs   5–10 ml
6–12 yrs   10–20 ml

Opioids

codeine	1.0 mg/kg im 4 hrly
morphine	0.1–0.2 mg/kg im 3–4 hrly
	0.5 mg/kg in 50 ml, 2 ml/hr by continuous iv infusion
	(= 0.02 mg/kg/hr), range 1–4 ml/hr
pethidine	1 mg/kg im 2–3 hrly

Sedation/paralysis in ICU

	Bolus (mg/kg)	Infusion (mg/kg/hr)
midazolam	0.5	0.1–0.4
fentanyl	0.001–0.003	0.001–0.004
morphine	0.1–0.2	0.02–0.04
atracurium	0.5	0.3–0.8
vecuronium	0.1	0.1–0.2
chloral hydrate	50 mg/kg via nasogastric tube, 6 hrly	

Antibiotics (parenteral doses)

	Dose	Comments
ampicillin	25 mg/kg, 6 hrly	
benzylpenicillin	25 mg/kg, 6 hrly	
cefotaxime	100–150 mg/kg/day in 2–4 doses; increase to 200 mg/kg/day in severe infection	Halve dose if GFR < 5 ml/min

PAEDIATRIC DRUGS (cont.)

	Dose	Comments
cefuroxime	200–240 mg/kg/day in 3 doses	12 hrly or once daily if GFR < 20 ml/min
erythromycin	25–50 mg/kg/day in 2–4 doses	Made up to 4 mg/ml (large volume)
flucloxacillin	25 mg/kg 6 hrly	
gentamicin	2 mg/kg 8 hrly	Monitor levels
sodium fusidate	2 mg/kg 8 hrly	Infusion over 6 hrs
trimethoprim	3 mg/kg 8 hrly	
vancomycin	10 mg/kg 6 hrly	Give over 60 mins; reduce dose in renal impairment, neonates and young infants

Fluid requirements
Maintenance crystalloid:

First 10 kg	4 ml/kg/hr	100 mls/kg/day
Second 10 kg	2 ml/kg/hr	50 mls/kg/day
Subsequent kg	1 ml/kg/hr	20 mls/kg/day

Compensate for pre-operative starvation with bolus of 10 ml/kg

LOCAL ANAESTHETICS

Drug	Onset	Relative potency	Relative duration	Toxicity	Physicochemical properties			Maximum safe dose mg/kg	
						pK$_B$	Partition co-efficient	% Protein binding	plain	With adrenaline
		(Lignocaine = 1)								
Amides										
Lignocaine	fast	1	1	medium	7.9	2.9	64	3	7
Bupivacaine	slow	4	3	medium	8.1	27.5	96	2	2
Prilocaine	fast	1	1.5	low	7.9	0.9	55	5	8
Esters										
Cocaine	fast	1	0.5	v. high	8.7	?	?	2	—
Amethocaine	slow	4	2	high	8.5	80	76	1.5	—

Systemic toxicity

CNS usually precedes CVS depression (?bupivacaine). Features include:

LOCAL ANAESTHETICS (cont.)

- numbness of tongue, circumoral tingling
- tinnitus
- lightheadedness
- visual disturbance
- 'strange sensation in head'
- tremor
- dysarthria, change in affect, drowsiness
- loss of consciousness → convulsions → apnoea
  (which together quickly lead to severe respiratory acidosis)

CVS effects on conduction, contractility and vascular tone:

- prolonged P-R interval, widening of QRS, AV dissociation
- bradyarrhythmias
- myocardial depression
- vasodilatation

Management of systemic toxicity

1) Avoid respiratory acidosis/hypoxaemia: Clear the airway and support respiration as necessary.

2) Specific treatment of convulsions and arrhythmias: 50–100 mg increments of thiopentone is probably treatment of choice for convulsions, although cardiorespiratory depression is possible. Muscle relaxants will control the muscular, but not cerebral, consequences of convulsions. Hypotension should be treated with leg elevation, iv fluids and vasopressors such as ephedrine and adrenaline. Bretyllium is regarded as the anti-arrhythmic drug of choice, although defibrillation remains the initial treatment for pulseless ventricular tachyarrhythmias.

Notes:

(i) Toxicity is related to plasma concentration, which in turn depends upon the dose, the rate of entry into circulation, the rate of metabolism/excretion and the intrinsic toxicity of the local anaesthetic used. Rates of absorption vary with the presence of vasoconstrictors, the tissue binding of the drug, and also the site of injection:
mucosal > intercostal/interpleural > nerve plexi > epidural > infiltration

(ii) The low toxicity of prilocaine is a result of extrahepatic metabolism. Its usefulness is limited by the risk of methaemoglobinaemia (caused by one its metabolites, *o*-toluidine), which is clinically significant when the dose exceeds 600 mg, (foetal Hb is particularly susceptible to this).

(iii) Bupivacaine: cardiac conduction delays may be first signs of toxicity and may lead to re-entrant phenomena and ventricular tachyarrhythmias. Reversing hypoxaemia and acidosis may be the key to successful resuscitation.

(iv) Anaphylactic reactions to the amides are very rare, and more commonly result from reactions to preservatives such as methylparahydroxybenzoate.

LOCAL ANAESTHETIC DOSAGE FOR SUBARACHNOID ANAESTHESIA

	Blockade to (ml)		
	L4	T10	T4
Lignocaine 5% (hyperbaric)	0.6–1.0	1.0–1.5	1.5–2.0
Bupivacaine 0.5% (isobaric)	2.0–3.0	2.5–3.5	—
Bupivacaine 0.5% (hyperbaric)	0.8–1.5	1.5–2.5	2.5–3.0

INTRAVENOUS REGIONAL ANAESTHESIA

Prilocaine is the drug of choice due to its low toxicity (bupivacaine must *never* be used). Suggested dosages as follows:

Weight (kg)	Dose (mg)	Volume of 0.5% solution (ml)
40	120	24
50	150	30
60	180	36
70	210	42

CARDIAC DRUGS

Inotropes/inoconstrictors/inodilators

Drugs	α_1	β_1	β_2	DA_1	PDEIII	Dose
Isoprenaline		+++	+			0.01–0.2 µg/kg/min
Adrenaline	+/++	+	+			0.02–0.2 µg/kg/min
Noradrenaline	+++	+				0.01–0.2 µg/kg/min
Dopamine 1–5 µg/kg/min 5–10 µg/kg/min > 10 µg/kg/min	 +	 + +	 + +	 ++ ++ ++		1–20 mg/kg/min
Dobutamine	0/+	+	+			1–25 µg/kg/min
Dopexamine		±	++++	+		0.5–6 µg/kg/min
Milrinone					+++	Loading: 50 µg/kg/min Infusion: 0.3–0.75 µg/kg/min
Enoximone					+++	Loading: 0.5–1 µg/kg/min Infusion: 5–20 µg/kg/min
Phenylephrine	+++					0.2–1 µg/kg/min

CARDIAC DRUGS (cont.)

Antiarrhythmic agents

Drug	Intravenous dose	Indications
Adenosine	3 mg over 2 secs into large vein; follow by 6 and 12 mg if ineffective after 1–2 mins	Rapid reversion to sinus rhythm from supraventricular tachycardias (including those associated with WPW). Also aids the diagnosis of broad and narrow complex tachycardias
Amiodarone	300 mg iv over 1 hr, followed by 900 mg over 23 hrs, then 600 mg daily for 7 days, then 200 mg daily	Tachycardias associated with WPW, and other supraventricular nodal and ventricular tachyarrhythmias unresponsive to other treatments
Bretylium tosylate	Loading dose 5–10 mg/kg over 10–20 mins followed 1–2 mg/min	VT or VF unresponsive to cardioversion ± lignocaine (may cause transient hypertension followed by hypotension)
Digoxin	Loading dose 0.75–1 mg over 2 hrs followed by maintenance of 63.5–500 μg daily according to renal function	Supraventricular tachycardias, (particularly AF) complete onset of action takes 1–2 hrs Therapeutic range 1–3 ng/ml
Esmolol	test dose of 5–10 mg iv loading dose 0.5 mg/kg over 2 mins followed by 50–200 μg/kg/min	Supraventricular tachycardia
Lignocaine	loading dose 1–1.5 mg/kg over 1 min maintenance 1–4 mg/min	Therapeutic level of 2–6 μg/ml First line treatment for dangerous ventricular ectopy (may cause hypotension)
Magnesium sulphate	loading dose: 8 mmol over 15 mins followed by 65 mmol over 24 hrs	Resistant ventricular arrhythmias
Verapamil	2.5 mg every 1–2 mins to a maximum of 10 mg. May be repeated every 2–4 hrs	Supraventricular tachycardia; may cause acute hypotension which can be reversed with 50–100 μg phenylephrine

Hypotensive agents

Vasodilators

Drug	Intravenous dose	Indications
Hydralazine	5–10 μg by slow iv injection infusion: 3–4 μg/kg/min reducing to 1–2 mg/kg/min	Arterial dilatation

31

A pocket reference to anaesthesia

CARDIAC DRUGS (cont.)		
Hypotensive agents		
Drug	**Dose**	**Action**
Vasodilators		
Sodium nitroprusside	Malignant hypertension 0.25–5 µg/kg/min Induced hypotension 0.25–1.5 µg/kg/min	Arterial and venous dilatation. Risk of CN⁻ toxicity > 8 µg/kg/min, with fatalities ≥ 15. Treat suspected CN⁻ toxicity with either: (i) dicobalt edetate 300 mg followed by 50 ml 50% glucose, or (ii) sodium nitrite 300 mg followed by 12.5 g sodiumthiosulphate
Glyceryl trinitrate	0.25–5 µg/kg/min	Venous dilatation
Isosorbide dinitrate	0.5–2.5 µg/kg/min	Venous dilatation
Phentolamine	Bolus: 0.5–5 mg Infusion: 0.5–20 µg/kg/min	α_1 blocker
ß-blockers		
Esmolol: Supraventricular tachycardia	Loading dose 500 µg/kg over 2 mins, followed by infusions of 50–200 µg/kg/min (see data sheet for details)	
perioperative hypertension	For immediate control, give bolus of 80 mgs over 15–30 secs, followed by infusion of 150–300 µg/kg/min according to response	
Labetalol	Bolus: 50 mg over 1 min, repeated every 5 mins to a maximum of 200 mg Infusion: 5–40 µg/kg/min	Combined α and ß blockade
Ganglion blockers		
Trimetaphan	5–30 µg/kg/min	
Others		
Clonidine	5–20 µg/min	Centrally acting α_2 agonist with analgesic and sedative properties
Nifedipine	10–20 mg sublingually or intranasally 8 hrly	Arterial dilatation

DRUG FORMULATION

Convenient administration of cardiac drug infusions can be achieved using one of the following regimens:
- prepare 3 x body weight (kg) in 50 ml; 1 ml/hr = 1 µg/kg/min
- use the nomogram shown below

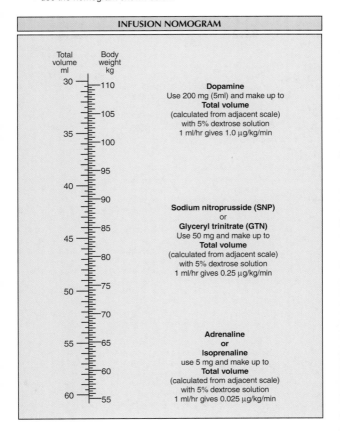

INFUSION NOMOGRAM

Total volume ml — Body weight kg

Dopamine
Use 200 mg (5ml) and make up to
Total volume
(calculated from adjacent scale)
with 5% dextrose solution
1 ml/hr gives 1.0 µg/kg/min

Sodium nitroprusside (SNP)
or
Glyceryl trinitrate (GTN)
Use 50 mg and make up to
Total volume
(calculated from adjacent scale)
with 5% dextrose solution
1 ml/hr gives 0.25 µg/kg/min

Adrenaline
or
Isoprenaline
use 5 mg and make up to
Total volume
(calculated from adjacent scale)
with 5% dextrose solution
1 ml/hr gives 0.025 µg/kg/min

COMPOSITION OF COMMONLY USED INTRAVENOUS FLUIDS

	Na^+ (mmol/l)	K^+ (mmol/l)	Cl^- (mmol/l)	lactate (mmol/l)	HCO_3^- (mmol/l)	Ca^{2+} (mmol/l)	Mg^{2+} (mmol/l)	dextrose (g/l)	pH	osmolality (mosml/l)
0.9% NaCl	154		154						5.0	308
0.45% NaCl	77	5	77						5.2	154
Hartmann's solution	131		112	29		1	1		6.5	280
4.3% dextrose/ 0.18% NaCl	31		31					43	4.5	300
5% dextrose								50	4.0	278
10% dextrose								100	4.0	523
8.4% NaHCO₃	1000				1000				8.0	2008
Mannitol 20%									6.0	1100
4.5% Human albumin solution	100–160	< 2	100–160		< 15 (citrate)				6.7–7.3	270–300
20% Human albumin solution	< 120	< 10	< 40		< 30 (citrate)					
Gelofusine 4%	154	0.4	125			0.4			7.4 ± 0.3	279
Hetastarch 6%	154		154						5.5	310
Haemaccel 3.5%	145	5.1	145			6.3			7.3 ± 0.3	
Dextran 70 in NaCl 0.9%	154		154						6.0	300
Dextran 70 in dextrose 5%								50	4.5	280

DRUG INTERACTIONS

The ability of one drug to interfere with the pharmacological activity of another may be pharmaceutical, pharmacokinetic or pharmacodynamic. Unless otherwise stated this table indicates the effect of administration of drug 1 on the pharmacological activity of drug 2.

Drug 1	Drug 2	Nature of interaction
Anti-hypertensive agents	Other hypotensive agents anaesthetics	enhanced hypotension
methyldopa, reserpine	d-tubocurare	hypotension
	NSAID	antagonism of hypotensive effect
α-blockers	halothane adrenaline	tachyarrhythmias (inhibition of α_2 receptors $\rightarrow$ increased neuronal NA release)
ß-blockers	histamine-releasing drugs	bronchospasm
	halothane	bradycardia myocardial depression
	morphine	$\uparrow$ effect ($\downarrow$ liver blood flow)
	insulin	hypoglycaemia
	sympathomimetics	severe hypertension (adrenoceptor upregulation)
trimetaphan	suxamethonium	prolongation of block (inhibition of pChE)
	non-depolarising relaxants	prolongation of block (inhibition of AChE)
	d-tubocurare	hypotension
ACE inhibitors	anaesthetics anxiolytics	hypotension
	diuretics	possible extreme hypotension
	NSAID	antagonism of hypotensive effect $\uparrow$ risk of renal failure and hyperkalaemia
	α-blockers	severe hypertension

DRUG INTERACTIONS (cont.)

Drug 1	Drug 2	Nature of interaction
Calcium channel blockers verapamil	halothane	bradycardia, AV delay, myocardial depression
	non-depolarising relaxants	enhanced effect
	dantrolene	myocardial depression hyperkalaemia
nifedipine	isoflurane	hypotension
	non-depolarising relaxants	enhanced effect
Antiarrhythmics	suxamethonium halothane	bradycardia
	2nd antiarrhythmic	hypotension
ß-blockers verapamil	halothane thiopentone	hypotension
quinidine propranolol	non-depolarising relaxants	prolongation of effect
quinidine procainamide	neostigmine	antagonism of cholinergic activity
	phenothiazines	ventricular arrhythmias
adenosine	theophylline	antagonism of antiarrhythmic effect
magnesium	hypotensive drugs	enhanced hypotension
	non-depolarising relaxants	prolonged effect
digoxin	Ca^{2+}	digoxin toxicity due to K^+ antagonism
	suxamethonium	bradycardia (both vagomimetic)
	K^+ losing diuretics	digoxin toxicity (hypokalaemia)
Antiasthma medication theophyllines	halothane catecholamines	tachyarrhythmias
	β_2 agonists	hypokalaemia
	adenosine	antagonism of antiarrhythmic effect

DRUG INTERACTIONS (cont.)

Drug 1	Drug 2	Nature of interaction
theophyllines (cont.)	ciprofloxacin erythromycin isoniazid	↑ plasma [theophylline]
	rifampicin	↓ plasma [theophylline]
	doxapram	CNS stimulation
ß₂ sympathomimetics	halothane	tachyarrhythmias
	catecholamines high-dose corticosteroids	hypokalaemia
	theophylline	hypokalaemia tachyarrhythmias
bambuterol	suxamethonium	prolonged effect
CNS drugs		
benzodiazepines	anaesthetics non-depolarising relaxants	additive effects
	erythromycin	inhibition of metabolism of midazolam
	cimetidine isoniazid omeprazole	inhibition of metabolism of diazepam
	rifampicin	enhanced metabolism of diazepam
fenfluramine	halothane	tachyarrhythmias
tricyclic antidepressants	adrenaline	x 3 ↑ effect
	noradrenaline	x 6 ↑ effect
	pancuronium ketamine	hypertension
	clonidine	antagonism of hypotensive effect
monoamine oxidase inhibitors	pethidine	excessive depressant or excitatory effects
	other opioids	possible increased sensitivity
	indirect sympathomimetics	life-threatening hypertension
	ketamine	hypertension

DRUG INTERACTIONS (cont.)

Drug 1	Drug 2	Nature of interaction
monoamine oxidase inhibitors (cont.)	myocardial depressants	possible hypotension
Lithium	metoclopramide	↑ extrapyramidal side effects
	NSAID	Li^+ toxicity (excretion)
	neostigmine	antagonism of cholinergic effect
	non-depolarising relaxants	prolongation of effect
	suxamethonium	delay and prolongation of effect
Phenothiazines	morphine	↑ effect (due to ↓ liver blood flow)
	anaesthetics	excessive sedation/ hypotension
	antihypertensive agents (particularly ACE inhibitors)	enhanced effect (α-blockade)
	quinidine procainamide	↑ risk of ventricular arrhythmias with drugs which prolong Q-T interval
	sulphonylureas	↑ hypoglycaemic effect
	desferrioxamine	avoid combination
	dopaminergics	antagonism
	Li^+	↑ risk of neurotoxicity and extrapyramidal side effects
	cimetidine	↑ effect of chlorpromazine
	metoclopramide	increased risk of extrapyramidal side effects
phenytoin	metronidazole trimethoprim	↑ plasma [phenytoin]
	rifampicin	↓ plasma [phenytoin]
	theophylline	↑ metabolism of theophylline
	sucralfate some enteral feeds	↓ GI metabolism of phenytoin

DRUG INTERACTIONS (cont.)		
Drug 1	**Drug 2**	**Nature of interaction**
Anti-Parkinson drugs		
amantidine	metoclopramide	extrapyramidal side effects
L-dopa	halothane	arrhythmias
	hypotensive agents	enhanced effect
	anxiolytics	occasional antagonism of diazepam, chlordiazepoxide
	metoclopramide domperidone	antagonism
selegiline	pethidine	hyperpyrexia, CNS toxicity
Cholinergics		
neostigmine pyridostigmine	quinidine, procainamide, aminoglycosides, lithium	antagonism of cholinergic action
neostigmine pyridostigmine ecothiopate eye drops	suxamethonium	prolongation of neuromuscular blockade
	non-depolarising relaxants	antagonism of neuromuscular blockade
Antibiotics		
aminoglycosides colistin clindamycin	neostigmine	antagonism of cholinergic effects
	non-depolarising relaxants	prolongation of action (presynaptic inhibition of ACh release)
	methoxyflurane	nephrotoxicity
aminoglycosides colistin vancomycin	loop diuretics	ototoxicity
amphotericin	aminoglycosides cyclosporin	nephrotoxicity
erythromycin	alfentanil midazolam theophylline	increased plasma levels of drug 2 (reduced metabolism)
erythromycin	digoxin	increased digoxin effect
azlocillin	non-depolarising relaxants	prolongation of action (presynaptic inhibition of ACh release)

DRUG INTERACTIONS (cont.)		
Drug 1	**Drug 2**	**Nature of interaction**
isoniazid	diazepam theophylline	increased effect (reduced metabolism)
4-quinolones	NSAID	↑ risk of convulsions
	theophylline	↑ plasma [theophylline]
	sucralfate	↓ GI absorption of ciprofloxacin
sulphonamides	procaine and related LA esters	inhibition of anti-bacterial activity
tetracycline	non-depolarising relaxants	prolongation of action (presynaptic inhibition of ACh release, ? Ca^{2+} chelation)
	methoxyflurane	nephrotoxicity
trimethoprim	procainamide	↑ plasma [procainamide]
vancomycin	aminoglycosides	↑ ototoxicity
Cytotoxic agents		
azathioprine cyclophosphamide thiotepa	suxamethonium	prolongation of effect
bleomycin	O_2	pulmonary O_2 toxicity
methotrexate (MTX)	NSAID	reduced excretion of MTX
Muscle relaxants		
dantrolene	verapamil	hyperkalaemia hypotension
suxamethonium	digoxin	bradyarrhythmias
	azathioprine bambuterol cyclophosphamide ecothiopate neostigmine procaine propanidid pyridostigmine thiotepa	prolonged action of suxamethonium

DRUG INTERACTIONS (cont.)

Drug 1	Drug 2	Nature of interaction
non-depolarising muscle relaxants	aminoglycosides azlocillin clindamycin colistin Mg^{2+} nifedipine procainamide propranolol quinidine verapamil	enhanced relaxation
NSAID		
	ACE inhibitors	renal failure, hyperkalaemia, antagonism of hypotensive effect
	Other NSAID	increased side effects
	4-quinolone antibiotics	↑ risk of convulsions
	anticoagulants	↑ risk of haemorrhage
	sulphonylureas	↑ hypoglycaemic effect
	loop diuretics	↑ risk of nephrotoxicity
	Li^+	reduced excretion → Li^+ toxicity
Opioids		
	metoclopramide	antagonism of gastric prokinetic effect
alfentanil	erythromycin	increased plasma [alfentanil]
dextropropoxyphene	carbamazepine	enhanced effect of carbamazepine
pethidine	MAOIs	CNS excitation or depression
	cimetidine	inhibition of metabolism of pethidine
Miscellaneous		
cimetidine	pethidine amiodarone flecainide lignocaine quinidine benzodiazepines chlormethiazole	increased plasma levels of drug 2 (reduced metabolism)

DRUG INTERACTIONS (cont.)

Drug 1	Drug 2	Nature of interaction
cimetidine (cont.)	propranolol labetalol theophylline	increased plasma levels of drug 2 (reduced metabolism)
cyclosporin	NSAID	nephrotoxicity
desferrioxamine	phenothiazines	manufacturers recommend avoidance
dipyridamole	adenosine	enhanced/prolonged effect of adenosine
disulfuram	chlordiazepoxide diazepam theophylline	inhibition of metabolism of drug 2
doxapram	sympathomimetics	hypertension
	theophylline	CNS stimulation
mifepristone	NSAID	manufacturer recommends avoidance of NSAID for 8–12 days after administration of mifepristone
omeprazole	diazepam	inhibition of metabolism of diazepam
sucralfate	ciprofloxacin phenytoin tetracycline	reduced GI absorption of drug 2
sulphonylureas	NSAID	enhanced hypoglycaemic effect
sympathomimetics	halothane cyclopropane	arrhythmias
	tricyclics	arrhythmias hypertension
	adrenergic neurone blockers	hypertension
	doxapram	CNS stimulation

FAILED INTUBATION

Immediate management

1. Administer 100% O_2, maintain airway and, if necessary, cricoid pressure.
2. SUMMON HELP.
3. Do not persist with attempts to intubate at expense of hypoxia and airway trauma.
4. Further management depends upon:
   - airway patency
   - risk of aspiration
   - need for intubation
   - need for general anaesthesia
   - nature of muscle relaxant used

Secondary management

1. Airway patent, stomach empty, non-depolarising relaxant given.
   a) Maintain oxygenation and anaesthesia.
   b) Continue to ventilate via face or laryngeal mask; attempt to intubate via blind nasal route, or by passing bougie or 6.5 mm endotracheal tube through correctly positioned laryngeal mask.
   c) If unsuccessful, consider whether the operation can be performed under:
      (i) local/regional anaesthesia – wake patient up.
      (ii) mask anaesthesia – reverse and convert.
   d) If GA/intubation required:
      (i) if procedure not essential – postpone operation.
      (ii) if essential, consider specialised intubating technique or tracheostomy under GA.
2. Airway obstructed.
   a) Administer 100% O_2, reposition head, insert oral or laryngeal airway.
   b) If no improvement, wake up, using transtracheal ventilation to maintain oxygenation:
      (i) ventilation via 10–14 g cannula through cricothyroid membrane (jet ventilation may lead to dangerous barotrauma if expiration through upper airway is not possible).
      (ii) surgical cricothyrotomy: 2–3 cm transverse incision in skin, identification and opening cricothyroid membrane and the passage of a 6 mm endotracheal tube in trachea with aid of dilators.
   c) If operation essential proceed either:
      (i) under local/regional anaesthesia.
      (ii) intubate or perform tracheostomy under local anaesthetic.
3. Full stomach (suxamethonium given).
   a) Administer 100% O_2, place head down in left lateral position, *maintaining cricoid pressure*.

FAILED INTUBATION (cont.)

b) Ventilate by face mask until spontaneous ventilation returns and wake patient up.

c) If surgery is essential, consider whether operation can be performed under:

    (i) local/regional anaesthesia – wake patient up and proceed.

    (ii) mask anaesthesia – wake patient up, pass wide-bore nasogastric tube, empty stomach and instill 30 ml Na citrate, then proceed under mask anaesthesia in head down (and, if possible, lateral) position.

d) If intubation required, wake patient up, empty stomach and consider specialized intubating technique or tracheostomy under local anaesthetic.

SEVERE BRONCHOSPASM AND ANAESTHESIA

Causes

- endotracheal tube in inadequately obtunded airway $\pm$ carinal/bronchial stimulation
- pre-existing asthma/COAD
- recent URTI
- children
- failed regional anaesthesia
- oral endoscopy, mediastinoscopy
- combination of histamine-releasing drugs and ß-blockers
- anaphylaxis
- pulmonary oedema

Management

1. General:

    a) Check patency/position of endotracheal tube.

    b) increase depth of anaesthesia with volatile agent (halothane traditionally, although beware combining this with ß-adrenergic agents in the presence of hypercarbia).

    c) increase F_iO_2.

2. Ventilation:

    a) Prolong expiratory time and reduce respiratory rate (6 breaths/min) in order to minimise gas trapping. Be prepared to tolerate respiratory acidosis. In extreme situations, manual compression of chest to aid expiration may be life-saving.

    b) Consider pneumothorax if a sudden deterioration in airway pressure or blood pressure occurs.

3. Pharmacological therapy:

If possible combine intravenous and nebulized treatment.

SEVERE BRONCHOSPASM AND ANAESTHESIA (cont.)

Intravenous treatment should include:

a)   Salbutamol 3–4 $\mu g/kg$ by slow bolus, followed by up to 50 $\mu g/min$ until spasm is broken or until heart rate 160 beats/min.

b)   Aminophylline (second line treatment):
     6 mg/kg by slow bolus (if not on oral theophylline) followed by 0.5 mg/kg/hr.

c)   Adrenaline is the treatment of choice in anaphylaxis.

d)   Hydrocortisone 200 mg 8 hrly.

e)   In refractory cases consider:
     • $MgSO_4$
     • ketamine
     • nebulised local anaesthetics
     • diethylether
     • cardiopulmonary bypass

ACID ASPIRATION

> 20 ml of gastric fluid pH < 2.5 may cause severe, acute pneumonitis.

Clinical features:
   • cyanosis
   • coughing, dyspnoea, tachypnoea, wheezing
   • fever, hypovolaemia, hypotension, metabolic acidosis
   • shadowing on chest X-ray (particularly R midzone)

Management

1.   If breathing spontaneously: place head down, on side, and wake up. If surgery is essential:
     a)   consider local/regional technique.
     b)   if GA required, pass nasogastric tube, empty stomach and instill 30 ml Na citrate, and proceed to rapid sequence induction.

2.   If paralysed: intubate trachea, place head down and apply suction. Proceed with surgery if condition allows. Pass nasogastric tube, empty stomach and instill 30 ml Na citrate. If respiratory function satisfactory, extubate patient when awake, on side and head down.

3.   General management:
     a)   administer 50% O_2.
     b)   ventilate only if clinically indicated – if pneumonitis is severe, may require high F_iO_2 plus PEEP.
     c)   perform rigid bronchoscopy if aspiration of particulate matter suspected.
     d)   treat bronchospasm with salbutamol 3–4 $\mu g/kg$ or aminophylline 6 mg/kg iv.
     e)   support circulation with fluids/inotropes as necessary.

ACID ASPIRATION (cont.)

f) chest X-ray.
g) chest physiotherapy.
h) antibiotics: controversial, although cover for *Staphylococcus, Pseudomonas* and anaerobes may be required.
i) steroids: not recommended.
j) monitor status with continuous pulse oximetry, regular blood – gas analysis and repeat chest X-ray.

MANAGEMENT OF DYSRHYTHMIAS DURING ANAESTHESIA

General principles:
- exclude hypoxia
- to treat hypercarbia, consider changing from halothane to enflurane or isoflurane and converting from spontaneous to controlled ventilation
- evaluate depth of anaesthesia
- consider checking serum K^+ and acid-base status

Atrial/ventricular ectopics
These are benign if they occur in isolation and the blood pressure is maintained. No specific therapy exists for the treatment of atrial ectopics but consider using lignocaine 1 mg/kg if ventricular ectopics are troublesome.

Supraventricular tachyarrhythmias
1. Sinus tachycardia (each QRS is preceded by normal P wave).
    a) treat cause, e.g. hypovolaemia, light anaesthesia.
2. Supraventricular tachycardia (SVT) (may be atrial or junctional in origin).
    a) If persistent, consider a therapeutic trial of adenosine 6–12 mg given rapidly into fast-flowing drip (will terminate junctional and temporarily slow atrial tachycardias [by slowing AV conduction]). This also allows differentiation between broad-complex SVT and ventricular tachy-cardia and treats Wolff-Parkinson-White syndrome SVT.
    b) If patient is hypotensive consider synchronized 50J DC cardioversion.
    c) If light anaesthesia is suspected, consider using a short acting ß-blocker, i.e. esmolol, and increase the depth of anaesthesia.
    d) Use verapamil 5 mg iv slowly (may cause hypotension, do not combine with ß-blockers).
3. Atrial fibrillation
    a) This is only a problem when the ventricular rate > 100 bpm.
    b) If it occurs in a patient with pre-operatively controlled AF, treat as for sinus tachycardia (although consider the possibility of hyperkalae-mic digoxin antagonism).
    c) If the patient was previously in sinus rhythm:
        i) consider synchronized DC shock (50J), particularly if the patient is hypotensive.

MANAGEMENT OF DYSRHYTHMIAS DURING ANAESTHESIA
(cont.)

    ii)   if light anaesthesia is suspected, use a short acting ß-blocker, i.e. esmolol, and increase depth of anaesthesia.

    iii) digoxin 500 µg over 5 mins or amiodarone 300 mg over 20 mins (the latter preferably into a central vein).

4. Atrial flutter

    a)   produces a saw-tooth pattern on ECG.

    b)   variable A-V block.

    c)   the use of adenosine may be diagnostically useful by slowing AV conduction and thereby revealing atrial flutter waves.

    Use synchronized DC shock (50J) or digoxin 500 µg over 5 mins.

5. Ventricular tachycardia

    This may be life-threatening and can be difficult to distinguish from broad-complex SVT. If no cardiac output is present, treat as for VF with unsynchronized DC shock (200J); if cardiac output is maintained exclude broad complex SVT (using adenosine) and treat with amiodarone 300 mg over 20 mins.

6. Heart block

    $1°$ and type I $2°$ heart block require no specific therapy. Type II heart block and complete heart block should be treated with atropine, isoprenaline (2 mg in 500 ml 5% dextrose, 4 µg/ml, starting at 1–2 ml/min) and temporary pacing (either intravenous, oesophageal or transthoracic).

PERIOPERATIVE HYPERTENSION

Common causes
- pain (including the full bladder)
- anxiety
- hypercarbia
- shivering
- existing hypertension

Rare causes
- malignant hyperthermia
- intracranial hypertension
- pre-eclampsia
- phaeochromocytoma

Management

1. Treat cause

2. If specific antihypertensive therapy required consider:

    a)   sublingual/intranasal nifedipine 10 mg PRN

    b)   hydralazine 10–20 mg

    c)   labetalol 20–50 mg (particularly if accompanied by tachycardia)

MANAGEMENT OF HIGH/TOTAL SPINAL BLOCKADE

This results from the inadvertant intrathecal injection of excessive quantities of local anaesthetic and may complicate epidural, intercostal, interpleural, paravertebral, brachial/cervical plexus or stellate ganglion blockade.

Total spinal is distinguished from high spinal blockade by the presence of respiratory failure (either due to phrenic nerve blockade or a direct action on the brainstem).

Features
- hypotension
- bradycardia
- respiratory failure
- loss of consciousness

Management

Restrict the cephalad spread of local anaesthetic by keeping the patient still and slightly head down (if hypobaric or isobaric solutions have been used). Support the circulation with fluids and inoconstrictors. Always give O_2 (have a low threshold for intubation and ventilatory support).

SEVERE ANAPHYLAXIS DURING ANAESTHESIA
(modified from Association of Anaesthetists' guidelines, 1990)

Features
- flushing, urticaria
- hypotension, tachycardia
- bronchospasm

Immediate management
1. Discontinue administration of the suspect drug.
2. SUMMON HELP.
3. Discontinue surgery and anaesthesia (if feasible).
4. Administer 100% O_2, and consider intubation and ventilation.
5. Give ADRENALINE in aliquots of 1–2 µg/kg to treat hypotension and bronchospasm (1 ml of 1:10 000 = 100 µg).
6. Start rapid intravascular volume expansion, preferably with colloid 10 mg/kg.
7. Consider external chest compression.

Secondary management
1. Bronchospasm: if unresponsive to adrenaline, consider SALBUTAMOL 250 µg iv loading dose, followed by 5–20 µg/min
   or TERBUTALINE 250–500 µg iv loading dose followed by 1.5 µg/min
   or AMINOPHYLLINE 6 mg/kg iv over 20 mins, followed by 0.5 mg/kg/hr.
2. Steroids: HYDROCORTISONE 500 mg
   or METHYLPREDNISOLONE 2 g iv.
3. Antihistamines: CHLORPHENIRAMINE 20 mg iv.

SEVERE ANAPHYLAXIS DURING ANAESTHESIA (cont.)

4. NaHCO$_3$ if acidosis is severe after 20 mins treatment.
5. Inoconstrictor infusions:
   - ADRENALINE 0.02–0.2 µg/kg/min
   - NORADRENALINE 0.02–0.2 µg/kg/min
     Make up as 0.03 mg/kg in 50 ml (1 ml/hr = 0.01 µg/kg/min)
     (These ranges are guidelines only, and larger doses may be required in the acute phase).
6. Check clotting screen, acid-base and blood gas status.
7. Take 5 ml blood into EDTA and plain tubes as soon as possible and repeat 3, 6 and 24 hrs later. Have samples centrifuged and stored at -20°C prior to characterisation of the immunological nature of the reaction.

POST-OPERATIVE RESPIRATORY INSUFFICIENCY

Causes

1. Pre-existing disease
   - malnutrition
   - myaesthenia gravis
   - myxoedema
   - myotonic dystrophy
   - severe sepsis
   - respiratory failure
   - heart failure

2. Anaesthetic causes
   - excessive anaesthesia (particularly in the absence of surgical stimulation/pain)
   - overdose of opioid
   - residual neuromuscular blockade
   - hypocarbia
   - hypothermia
   - acid-base and electrolyte disturbance – in particular the vicious circle of respiratory acidosis potentiating the effects of residual neuromuscular blockade

Management

1. Assess depth of anaesthesia, residual neuromuscular blockade and possibility of narcotic overdose, and treat as appropriate with:
   a) neostigmine and anticholinergic (do not exceed 5 mg neostigmine).
   b) naloxone 100 µg boluses (up to 400 µg initially).
2. If no immediate response occurs, check arterial blood gases, temperature and chest X-ray.
3. If intubated, continue to ventilate to normocarbia.
4. If extubated, give O$_2$ by face mask but have a low threshold for re-intubation unless you are sure the problem can be quickly corrected. Only use respiratory stimulants such as doxapram if you are confident that the problem is a short term one, e.g. residual anaesthesia.

AIR (OR GAS) EMBOLISM

Causes:

1. Surgical: operations in which open veins are above level of heart; neurosurgery (particularly sitting position), breast surgery, thoracic surgery, pelvic surgery.

2. Diagnostic/therapeutic injections of gas: laparoscopy, thoracoscopy, injection into joints.

3. Accidental entry during intravenous techniques, e.g. during insertion of central lines.

Pathophysiology:

Paradoxical arterial embolism: < 1 ml sufficient to occlude major cerebral or coronary artery.

Venous air embolism (VAE): 0.4 ml/kg/min causes 'multiple pulmonary embolism' syndrome, with increased pulmonary arterial pressures, gas exchange defects and right sided heart failure. 0.5–1 ml/kg as rapid bolus is sufficient to completely occupy right ventricle and thereby abolish cardiac output.

Diagnosis of VAE:

- visible/audible entry of air
- irregular, gasping respiration
- tachyarrhythmias
- hypotension
- mill wheel murmur
- cardiac arrest

Detection of VAE:

• transoesophageal echo/precordial Doppler	0.02 ml/kg/min
• capnography (demonstrates a fall in $P_{ET}CO_2$)	0.4 ml/kg/min
• increased pulmonary artery pressures	0.4 ml/kg/min
• hypotension, high CVP	0.7 ml/kg/min
• mill wheel murmur, CVS collapse	1.7 ml/kg/min

Management:

1. Inform surgeon, compress entry veins and swamp site with saline; discontinue N_2O (it expands the embolus) and give 100% O_2; lower entry site to below the level of the heart.

2. If hypotensive:

    (i)   place 15° head down on right side (Durant position) to limit further entry of air into heart (will make CPR difficult).

    (ii) aspirate air from CVP line or, if desperate, by needle puncture of RV.

    (iii) support circulation with fluids and inotropes.

PERIOPERATIVE PULMONARY OEDEMA

$$f \propto [(P_c - P_i) - \sigma(\pi_c - \pi_i)]$$

f = fluid flux across pulmonary capillary endothelium
$P_c - P_i$ = hydrostatic pressure gradient
$\pi_c - \pi_i$ = oncotic pressure gradient
σ = reflection coefficient (normal 0.7 → 0 in acute lung injury)

Aetiology

1. Hydrostatic – increased Pc: *low cardiac output state ± ECG signs of ischaemia, high filling pressure.*

   a) ↑ LVEDP
      - fluid overload – including increased venous return in Trendelenburg or lithotomy position
      - LV failure – cardiomyopathy, ischaemia/infarction, myocardial depressant drugs, arrhythmias
      - reduced LV compliance – tamponade, pericarditis, LV hypertrophy

   b) ↑ LAP
      - mitral valve disease, external compression

   c) ↑ pulmonary venous pressure
      - atrial myxoma, thrombus, venous constriction

   d) ↑ pulmonary arterial pressure
      - pulmonary hypertension, hyperperfusion (e.g. after pneumonectomy)

2. Increased capillary membrane permeability (reduced σ): *high output state ± signs of hypovolaemia, low filling pressures.*
   - acid aspiration
   - severe sepsis
   - fat/gas/amniotic fluid embolism
   - toxic gas inhalation
   - acute pancreatitis
   - lung contusion
   - anaphylaxis

3. Mixed
   - neurogenic
   - lung re-expansion following relief of upper airway obstruction

Management

1. ↑ F_iO_2
   a) add CPAP, IPPV + PEEP as necessary.
   b) have low threshold for use of pulmonary artery catheter.

PERIOPERATIVE PULMONARY OEDEMA (cont.)

Hydrostatic

Aim: reduce P_c

diuretics/inotropes/
vasodilatation
mask CPAP or ventilation
if necessary

Membrane

Aim: increase P_i

IPPV + PEEP are mainstay of
support
avoid frequent suction
(nullifies PEEP and worsens
alveolar flooding) treat
hypovolaemia with cautious
colloid infusion; avoid diuretics

MALIGNANT HYPERTHERMIA

Clinical Presentation

- Masseter spasm or generalized muscle rigidity
- Unexplained desaturation, tachycardia, tachypnoea
- Unstable cardiac rhythm
- Fever, sweating, rapid temperature rise ($2°C/hr$)
- Unexplained rise of end-tidal CO_2
- Unexplained myoglobinuria

Associated laboratory abnormalities

- Metabolic and respiratory acidosis
- Hyperkalaemia
- Marked increase in creatinine kinase over 24 hrs
- Myoglobinuria (first specimen of urine)
- Evidence of disseminated intravascular coagulation

Treatment protocol

1) Discontinue inhalational agents; convert to malignant hyperthermia (MH) safe technique and use vapour-free machine and circuit.

2) Terminate surgery as soon as possible.

3) Monitor ECG, core and peripheral temperature, end-tidal CO_2, CVP, arterial pressure, urine output, arterial blood gases, urea and electrolytes, creatinine kinase and clotting screen.

4) Cool actively with tepid sponging, fanning, cool iv and nasogastric fluids. Avoid severe vasoconstriction which will impede heat loss.

5) Hyperventilate (3 x minute volume) with 100% O_2.

6) Dantrolene 1 mg/kg rapidly iv (up to 10 mg/kg as required, normally approximately 2.5 mg/kg).

7) Treat acidosis with 1.5 ml/kg 8.4% $NaHCO_3$ i.v. stat.

8) Treat hyperkalaemia with 50 mls 50% dextrose + 10 units of insulin; if uncontrolled, consider ion exchange resins and even dialysis.

9) Promote urine output with iv fluids; consider mannitol 1 g/kg (remember that 20 mg vial of dantrolene contains 3 g mannitol).

MALIGNANT HYPERTHERMIA (cont.)

10) Monitor temperature for 24–48 hrs (occasional spikes of temperature occur after the initial episode, but a persisting pyrexia suggests another cause).

11) Repeat creatinine kinase estimation after 24 hrs.

12) Arrange elective muscle biopsy (if a child, the parents will require biopsy).

Anaesthesia for MH susceptible patients

1. Drugs considered safe in MH
   - benzodiazepines
   - thiopentone, propofol (and other IV induction agents)
   - N_2O
   - fentanyl (and other opioids)
   - NSAID
   - atracurium, vecuronium
   - droperidol

2. Drugs to avoid in MH

Suxamethonium and **all** the anaesthetic vapours are absolutely contraindicated. Although less clear, it is probably wise to avoid tricyclics, MAOIs and phenothiazines.

Monitoring should include:

Non-invasive BP, ECG, S_aO_2, end-tidal CO_2, core temperature (which should commence 2–3 hrs before surgery and continue for several hrs post-operatively).

The anaesthetic machine and circuits should be vapour free. Pre-treatment with dantrolene is not recommended, but should be immediately available in theatre.

CYANOSIS DURING ANAESTHESIA

Clinical detection is a notoriously unreliably clinical sign and requires the presence of > 5 g/dl of deoxyhaemoglobin.

Common causes:
- misplaced endotracheal tube (ETT)
- disconnection of gas delivery system
- obstruction (of airway or ETT)
- O_2 supply failure
- cardiac arrest

1. Chest problems
   - severe bronchospasm
   - pneumothorax
   - haemothorax
   - pulmonary oedema
2. Circulation problems
   - anaphylaxis
   - low cardiac output states
   - pulmonary embolism – clot, gas, amniotic fluid, fat
3. O_2 supply failure
   - pipeline problem
   - machine problem
   - cylinder exhaustion
   - breathing circuit problem
4. ETT problems
   - oesophageal, pharyngeal, endobronchial intubation
   - kinked (perform laryngoscopy)
   - obstruction (pass bougie, suction catheter)
5. If in doubt:
   - ventilate manually with air or O_2 from cylinder
   - change ETT
   - change anaesthetic machine and use cylinder O_2 supply

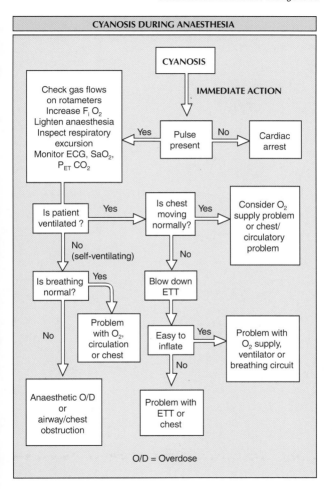

CYANOSIS DURING ANAESTHESIA

CYANOSIS

IMMEDIATE ACTION

Check gas flows on rotameters
Increase $F_i O_2$
Lighten anaesthesia
Inspect respiratory excursion
Monitor ECG, SaO_2, $P_{ET} CO_2$

Pulse present — **Yes** / **No** → Cardiac arrest

Is patient ventilated? — **Yes** → Is chest moving normally? — **Yes** → Consider O_2 supply problem or chest/circulatory problem

No (self-ventilating)

Is breathing normal? — **Yes** → Problem with O_2, circulation or chest

No → Is chest moving normally? — **No** → Blow down ETT

Easy to inflate — **Yes** → Problem with O_2 supply, ventilator or breathing circuit

No → Problem with ETT or chest

Anaesthetic O/D or airway/chest obstruction

O/D = Overdose

PERIOPERATIVE MANAGEMENT OF DIABETES MELLITUS

Management depends upon the nature and effectiveness of current diabetic control, together with the type of surgery planned.

Aims of management (in order of priority) are to avoid:

- Hypoglycaemia (particularly during anaesthesia)
- Ketoacidosis
- Hyperglycaemia, osmotic diuresis and dehydration

Procedures in which cerebral ischaemia is possible (such as neurosurgery carotid endarterectomy and cardiac surgery) demand more precise blood sugar control.

The most important factor in good peri-operative glycaemic control is the frequent measurement of blood glucose by well-trained staff.

DIABETES MANAGEMENT GUIDELINES			
	Pre-operatively	**Day of operation**	**Post-operatively**
Diet controlled	Check random blood sugar		
Well controlled	Treat as normal	Treat as normal	Monitor: may become insulin-dependent following major surgery
Poorly controlled	Postpone and control: if urgent and for major surgery start insulin/glucose regimen		
Oral hypoglycaemics	Check random blood sugar, U+Es	Check fasting blood sugar, U+Es	
Well controlled	Stop sulphonylureas one half life prior to surgery. Stop metformin 24 hrs pre-op due to risk of lactic acidosis	Minor surgery: omit oral agent on morning of operation – restart with first meal. Major surgery: omit oral agent on morning of operation and treat as poorly controlled (see below)	
Poorly controlled	Start tds soluble insulin and delay surgery. If urgent start iv insulin/glucose infusion	Treat as insulin-dependent peri- and post-op, resuming oral agents when post-op insulin requirements < 20 units/day	

DIABETES MANAGEMENT GUIDELINES (cont.)			
	Pre-operatively	**Day of operation**	**Post-operatively**
Insulin-dependent	Check 24hr blood sugar profile, U+Es, urinary ketones	No sc insulin in morning: check fasting blood sugar, U+Es. Establish GIK regimen early in the day and check blood sugar 2 hrly pre-op and half hrly intra-op	Check blood sugar 2–4 hrly Minor surgery: replace GIK regimen with tds sc soluble insulin when oral intake resumed
Well controlled	Stop long-acting insulin/halve dose of intermediate acting insulin on evening prior to surgery		Major surgery: replace GIK regimen with separate glucose/insulin infusions if delayed post-op recovery anticipated. Convert to tds sc insulin when oral intake resumed
Poorly controlled	Delay surgery and convert to tds soluble insulin regimen. If urgent start iv insulin/glucose infusion		In both cases, restart normal insulin when requirements stable
GIK = glucose–insulin–potassium sc = subcutaneous			

Insulin preparations			
	Subcutaneous onset of action (hrs)	**Maximum effect (hrs)**	**Duration of action (hrs)**
Short acting e.g. neutral insulins such as actrapid, humilin S	0.5–1	2–4	< 12
Intermediate, e.g. isophane insulin	1–2	3–8	16–18
Long-acting, e.g. insulin lente, protamine zinc insulin	> 2	8–12	20–40

DIABETES MANAGEMENT GUIDELINES (cont.)

Glucose-insulin-potassium (GIK) regimen

100 ml/hr of 500 ml 10% dextrose to which soluble insulin and potassium have been added according to the following scales:

Blood sugar (mmol/l)	Units insulin/500 ml 10% dextrose
< 5	5
5–10	10
10–20	15
> 20	20

Plasma K$^+$ (mmol/l)	Added KCl/500 ml 10% dextrose
< 3	20 mmol
3–5	10 mmol
> 5	nil

Check potassium pre- and post-operatively and then daily whilst the infusion continues. Monitor blood glucose 1–2 hrly (wasteful for prolonged post-operative use).

Sliding scale insulin infusion

(a) IV fluid. Give 100 ml/hr 10% dextrose, although prolonged use may require smaller volumes of more concentrated dextrose solutions to allow replacement of salt losses.

(b) Potassium. Add 20 mmol KCl per litre of 10% dextrose: measure potassium pre- and post-operatively and then daily whilst on regimen. Increase to 30 mmol/l if K$^+$ < 4 and omit if K$^+$ > 5 mmol/l

(c) Insulin infusion: 50 units soluble insulin in in 50 ml saline (i.e. 1 unit/ml). Adjust insulin infusion according to blood sugar measured 1–2 hrly.

Blood sugar (mmol/l)	Units insulin/hr
< 4	0
4.1–9	1
9.1–11	2
11.1–17	3
17.1–28	4
> 28	6 (and review infusion)

Permits easier and more economic manipulation of blood glucose post-operatively, but allows insulin to be administered without concomitant dextrose infusion (and therefore risks hypoglycaemia).

Half-lives of oral hypoglycaemic agents			
Acetolexamide	3 hrs	Glipizide	3–6 hrs
Chlorpropamide	25–42 hrs (mean 33)	Gliquidone	3 hrs
Glibenclamide	8–10 hrs	Tolbutamide	6 hrs
Gliclazide	10–15 hrs	Metformin	18 hrs

ANAESTHESIA AND PORPHYRIA

Problems arise principally with the acute variants of this condition (which include Acute Intermittent, Variegate and Hereditary Coproporphyria) and result from the drug-mediated induction of enzymes which generate increased quantities of porphyrin metabolites. Acute attacks usually resolve completely but can be fatal. Features include:

- initial hypertension and tachycardia, although left ventricular failure and hypotension may ensue
- abdominal pain, vomiting
- peripheral neuropathy, upper motor neurone disorders, urinary retention, cranial nerve palsies, inappropriate secretion of ADH
- fever and leucocytosis

Precipitants:
- drugs (see table below)
- starvation
- infections (and possibly the antibiotics used to treat it)
- pregnancy

ANAESTHETIC DRUGS AND PORPHYRIA		
	Precipitants	**Drugs considered safe**
Induction agents	thiopentone, methohexitone, etomidate	propofol, ketamine
Inhalational agents	halothane, enflurane	isoflurane
Muscle relaxants	alcuronium	suxamethonium, atracurium, vecuronium
Analgesics	dextropropoxyphene, pentazocine, diclofenac, mefenamic acid	morphine, diamorphine, codeine, pethidine, dihydrocodeine
Local anaesthetics	lignocaine, prilocaine, cocaine	bupivacaine
Anti-emetics	metoclopramide	prochlorperazine, domperidone
Antacids	AL-containing agents	ranitidine, sodium citrate
Vasopressors		ephedrine, adrenaline, methoxamine
Antiepileptics		diazepam (with caution)
Miscellaneous	hyoscine, theophylline	

ANAESTHESIA AND SICKLE CELL DISEASE

Sickle cell disease is an inherited disorder which ranges from a benign heterozygous condition (HbAS, sickle cell trait) to the sickle cell disease syndromes. The latter spectrum of the disorder, in which either the homozygous form (HbSS) or combination with other Hb variants (HbSC, HbSD, HbSE, HbSß-thalassaemia) exist, can lead to life-threatening clinical problems.

Distribution and incidence

Negro populations in central Africa, West Indies and North America; lower incidence in the Indian subcontinent and Mediterranean regions.

Pathophysiology

HbS differs from HbA by the substitution of valine for glutamic acid at position 6 of the ß-chain of the globin molecule. This results in a Hb molecule which, although soluble when oxygenated, crystallises out of solution when deoxygenated to distort erythrocytes and give them their characteristic sickle shape. Sickled erythrocytes obstruct the microcirculation and thereby lead to tissue ischaemia/infarction.

The principal cause of sickling is a reduction in tissue O_2 tension. Crises are therefore induced by hypoxia, hypothermia, dehydration, acidosis and infection. In patients with the sickle cell trait, 20–40% of the total Hb is HbS; sickling does not occur significantly until the tissue PO_2 has fallen to ≤ 2.5 kPa. In HbSS, in contrast, 95–98% of Hb is HbS and sickling occurs at tissue PO_2 of ≤ 5.5 kPa.

Diagnosis

Hb electrophoresis is the definitive investigation. The sickledex test simply identifies the presence of HbS and does not, therefore, distinguish between the sickle cell trait and the disease. Although a positive sickledex test and normal Hb concentration in an adult make HbSS unlikely, other variants such as HbSC are possible. This is important because these patients are susceptible to peri-operative sickling crises. In the absence of a full haematological assessment, therefore, all patients with a positive sickledex test should be considered to be at risk of peri-operative infarctive crises.

Anaesthetic management of sickle cell trait (HbAS)

Although these patients may have mild anaemia, their Hb concentration is usually normal. Despite the risk of peri-operatively sickling being small, it is sensible to treat with care. Management should include:

- Maintenance of oxygenation
- Prevention of hypothermia
- Prevention of dehydration
- Avoidance of prolonged use of tourniquets
- For patients with high HbS levels undergoing major procedures pre-operative exchange transfusion should be considered

ANAESTHESIA AND SICKLE CELL DISEASE (cont.)

Anaesthetic management of sickle cell disease
(HbSS, HbSC, HbS ß- thalassaemia)

Pre-existing problems include anaemia (Hb 5–8 g/dl), cor pulmonale due to recurrent chest infections and pulmonary emboli, renal impairment, iron overload, cerebrovascular disease and increased susceptibility to bacterial infection (particularly streptococci and coliforms) because of asplenism.

Pre-operative exchange transfusion is usually required, and should aim to bring the Hb concentration to approximately 10 g/dl and HbA level to $\geq$ 50%. Peri-operative alkalization, designed to inhibit sickling by raising blood pH, is of unproven value. General measures include maintenance of body temperature, hydration and oxygenation at all times. Meticulous attention should be paid to positioning on the operating table to avoid venous stasis. Tourniquets should only be used if absolutely necessary. Monitoring of mixed venous O_2 saturation may be of value in major surgery.

Post-operative care should be provided in a high dependency setting. Adequate analgesia (to facilitate early mobilisation) should be provided whenever possible, together with prophylactic antibiotics to reduce the incidence of pulmonary sepsis. Sickling crises are most likely to occur in the early post-operative period and may be heralded by vague aches and pains. Anticoagulation should be considered if marrow infarction (suggested by bone pain) develops.

ANAESTHESIA AND PACEMAKERS

Pre-operative considerations:

1. The patient is likely to have significant CVS disease (50% ischaemic heart disease, 20% hypertension, 10% diabetes).
2. Evaluation of pacemaker function: check type and date of last check-up. In particular check manufacturer's literature regarding the response of the pacemaker to diathermy (most modern ones are not affected). Determine site of pacemaker, and whether a magnet is available to convert the 'on-demand' to 'fixed rate'. If fixed rate, > 10% reduction below set rate suggests power source depletion. If demand pacemaker, check the response to carotid massage or Valsalva manouevre.
3. Consider antibiotic prophylaxis against endocarditis.

Intra-operative considerations:

1. Diathermy. The principle problem is the possibility of sensing diathermy currents by the pacemaker, which may then switch off (I type) or trigger (T type) the pacing mechanism (the latter being particularly dangerous).
   - If possible, avoid diathermy
   - If necessary, use bipolar rather than unipolar diathermy
   - If unipolar diathermy has to be used, place diathermy earthing plate as far away from the pacemaker as possible
   - If diathermy-induced inhibition is a problem, use magnet to convert from 'on-demand' to 'fixed' mode

2. Use diathermy-immune pulse rate monitoring.
3. Patients treated with ventricular pacing devices are particularly sensitive to volume depletion due to the loss of active atrial filling.
4. Danger of microshock with temporary pacing wires.
5. Central venous and pulmonary artery catheterisation may dislodge pacing wires, particularly if inserted within the last six weeks.
6. Be ready to manage pacemaker failure with an isoprenaline infusion.
7. Post-operatively inform pacemaker clinic if diathermy has been used to enable the pacemaker programming to be checked.

ANAESTHESIA AND PACEMAKERS

Five letter coding system of pacemaker classification	
1st letter: chamber being paced	A — atrium V — ventricle D — dual chamber
2nd letter: chamber being sensed	A — atrium V — ventricle D — dual chamber
3rd letter: sensing response	I — inhibited T — triggered D — dual response
4th letter: programmability	O — none P — simple M — multi-programmable R — adaptive rate pacing
5th letter: tachyarrhythmic functions	O — none P — pacing S — DC shock for VT, VF

Indications for temporary pacing pre-operatively

Criteria are continuously changing (consult a cardiologist if possible) but currently include:

1. Right bundle branch block and left posterior hemiblock (particularly if symptomatic or combined with $1°$ heart block)
2. Left bundle branch block and $1°$ heart block
3. Mobitz Type I $2°$ heart block if > 3:1 A–V conduction failure
4. Mobitz Type II $2°$ heart block
5. Third degree heart block
6. Symptomatic bradycardic syndromes, e.g. sinus pause, sick sinus syndrome
7. Congenital complete heart block (particularly if unresponsive to anticholinergics)

PERIOPERATIVE MANAGEMENT OF HAEMOPHILIA A

Haemophilia A is an X-linked factor VIII deficiency with variable expression. The principal problem is *delayed bleeding from large vessels* with typically a prolonged APTT with normal PTR/TT.

Principles of management

1. Factor VIII replacement: the aim is to keep plasma factor VIII activity ≥100–150% normal, and particularly to avoid level <50%. Replacement therapy is started pre-operatively and continued for 7–10 days post-operatively. The plasma half life of factor VIII concentrate means that doses are required 8–12 hrly.

   a) Pre-operatively, measure plasma factor VIII levels, together with any factor VIII antagonist activity. Calculate (in conjunction with a haematologist) the dose of factor VIII necessary to elevate levels ≥ 100% of normal, which will depend upon:
      • intrinsic plasma factor VIII activity
      • presence of antagonists
      • body weight
      • intrinsic activity of the factor VIII concentrate available

   If factor VIII concentrate is not available during an emergency, give 20 ml/kg fresh frozed plasma (FFP). DDAVP, 0.3 μg/kg iv over 15 mins in 20 ml NaCl may increase efficacy of endogenous factor VIII.

   b) Post-operatively, monitor factor VIII activity and calculate the dose and dosage interval for post-operative replacement.

2. Other problems and considerations

   a) Due to risk of haemorrhage, avoid:
      • im injections
      • regional anaesthetic techniques
      • unnecessary intubation (particularly via nasal route)
      • unnecessary arterial sampling
      • subclavian/internal jugular venous cannulation
        (femoral vein is central vein of choice)
      • anti-platelet drugs

   b) Care with positioning
      (many patients have joint disease due to haemarthroses)

   c) Up to 80% of haemophiliacs treated before 1985 are expected to be HIV positive (there is also an increased incidence of hepatitis B).

MYOTONIC DYSTROPHY

Myotonic dystrophy is an autosomal dominant condition which is also known as Steinert's disease or myotonia atrophica. The onset of symptoms occurs in early adult life and leads to death from respiratory/cardiac failure by 60 years of age.

Clinical features

- Classic triad of frontal baldness, cataracts and mental retardation
- Skeletal muscle atrophy leading to weakness of facial, neck, respiratory and distal musculature
- Failure of muscle relaxation (myotonia) following voluntary or induced contraction (e.g. diathermy, shivering, transcutaneous nerve stimulation)
- Pharyngeal muscle weakness which may lead to aspiration
- Impaired smooth muscle function which can cause impaired gastric emptying
- Myotonic dystrophy is associated with a significant incidence of sudden cardiac death; problems include 1° heart block (not reversed by anticholinergics), mitral valve prolapse (20%), cardiomyopathy
- Endocrine problems: gonadal atrophy, diabetes mellitus, hypothyroidism and adrenal insufficiency
- Central sleep apnoea
- Symptoms deteriorate during pregnancy (uterine atony)

Anaesthetic considerations

- Continue pre-operative medication (usually phenytoin, quinine or procainamide)
- Cardiovascular disease may require pre-operative pacing and the use of pulmonary artery flotation catheter
- Risk of post-operative chest infections/respiratory failure makes regional techniques attractive
- May require steroid supplements
- Sensitive to respiratory depressants such as benzodiazepines, opioids and barbiturates
- 50% of patients will develop life-threatening myotonia following the use of suxamethonium (non-depolarising relaxants are safe)
- Post-operative shivering may induce myotonic crisis

Management of myotonia

- Deepen general anaesthesia using respiratory support
- Non-depolarising relaxants are unlikely to be effective
- The efficacy of dantrolene remains unclear
- Intramuscular lignocaine or procaine can be of value
- Intrauterine bupivacaine has been used to treat uterine atony

ANAESTHETIC MANAGEMENT OF MYASTHENIA GRAVIS

Myasthenia gravis is an autoimmune-mediated disorder of neuromuscular transmission. It may be associated with thymoma, other autoimmune disorders such as SLE or rheumatoid arthritis, pernicious anaemia, thyrotoxicosis or, rarely, cardiomyopathy.

Clinical features

- Fatigue-induced initially, weakness of ocular, facial and bulbar muscles initially, later extending to respiratory and limb musculature
- Bulbar palsy may lead to aspiration and recurrent chest infections
- EMG shows reduced single twitch height and fade with tetanic or train of four stimulation
- Medical treatment includes the use of anticholinesterases (± anticholinergics), steroids, azathioprine, cyclosporin and ephedrine. Plasmapheresis is used in severe cases
- Deterioration may be due to disease progression, intercurrent infection, or under- or over-dosage with anticholinesterase

Anaesthetic management

1. Pre-operative considerations

   a) Carefully assess respiratory function and airway reflexes.

   b) Warn about the potential need for post-operative ventilation and discuss regional anaesthesia/analgesia. Omit pre-operative anticholinesterases if ventilation is planned, but continue if a regional technique or spontaneous ventilation is likely.

2. Intra-operative considerations

   a) Use a local or regional technique whenever possible (although thoracic blocks may compromise respiratory function). Intubation and ventilation is necessary for general anaesthesia except for patients with mild disease (and normal respiratory function) undergoing minor surgery.

   b) The response to suxamethonium is unpredictable (both resistance and sensitivity have been reported), although it should be used if the airway is at risk. Recent plasmapheresis may have depleted plasma cholinesterase activity. Patients may be extremely sensitive to non-depolarising relaxants which, if used at all, should be given in doses of 10–20% of normal (monitoring of neuromuscular blockade is mandatory). Atracurium has obvious attractions. Neuromuscular blockade should never be reversed, and factors enhancing blockade (e.g. hypothermia, hypokalaemia, aminoglycosides) avoided.

3. Post-operative considerations

   a) Elective ventilation is often required.

   b) Because anticholinesterase requirements may fall post-operatively, gradually increase the dose (either iv or via nasogastric tube) until muscle power and respiratory function is acceptable.

ANAESTHESIA AND MONOAMINE OXIDASE INHIBITORS (MAOI)

MAOIs include phenelzine, isocarboxazid, tranylcypromine

Irreversible inhibition of CNS and peripheral monoamine oxidase leads to increased levels of neuronal monoamine neurotransmitters (e.g. noradrenaline). Displacement of enhanced levels of neurotransmitters leads to life threatening CVS instability and CNS dysfunction. Anaesthetic problems with concurrent MAOI therapy are anecdotal, unpredictable and seem to occur in only a minority of patients receiving such therapy. Current opinion is that these drugs **need not be** stopped prior to surgery provided that anaesthesia is conducted carefully and certain drugs are avoided, thereby avoiding the potentially serious psychiatric consequences of MAOI discontinuation. Conversion to the shorter acting, reversible MAO–A inhibitor moclobemide 2–3 weeks before surgery, which is then stopped 24 hrs pre-operatively, is another option.

Peri-operative management

1. Premedication: Adequate premedication with a benzodiazepine will reduce both anxiety and sympathetic discharge, thereby helping to avoid CVS instability
2. Opioids: Pethidine is a major problem, *and must not be given.* Two potentially life-threatening reactions may occur:
   (a) Excitatory – agitation, hypertension, hyperpyrexia, headache, coma and convulsions (possibly due to raised 5-HT levels in CNS).
   (b) Depressive – respiratory depression, hypotension and coma (possibly due to inhibition of hepatic metabolism).
   Morphine and fentanyl appear much less likely to cause problems, although some advocate the use of test doses (e.g. 1–2 mg morphine).
3. Intravenous and inhalational anaesthetics: Occasional reports of problems with thiopentone. Other agents appear to be safe, although it would seem prudent to avoid ketamine.
4. Local anaesthetics: Avoid cocaine; the use of other agents is considered safe as are added vasoconstrictors (e.g. adrenaline).
5. Sympathomimetic agents: Indirect sympathomimetics such as ephedrine are *absolutely contraindicated,* as they cause life-threatening hypertensive crises following the displacement of enhanced levels of stored catecholamines. Directly acting agents are safer, although they may have an enhanced effect and should be initiated at one-third of their usual dose.
6. Monitoring: Have a low threshold for invasive blood pressure monitoring.

PERIOPERATIVE STEROID REPLACEMENT

While the normal physiological secretion of glucocorticoids from the adrenal cortex is approximately 30 mg of cortisol per day, this can rise to 200–400 mg as part of the stress response to major surgery. Long-term corticosteroid therapy can suppress this adrenocortical response to trauma. While most patients with suppressed adrenocortical function will have no peri-operative cardiovascular problems, a minority may develop life-threatening hypotension, hyponatraemia and hyperkalaemia if peri-operative steroid supplements are not given.

Who requires supplements

1. In the absence of biochemical information regarding the responsiveness of the adrenal cortex, all patients on steroids, or who have taken them within the last twelve months (either inhaled, systemic or topical) should be considered to be at risk, although this will be greater when the daily oral intake of prednisolone is ≥ 7.5 mg
2. Patients with deficient glucocorticoid production:
   - Adrenal insufficiency (primary or secondary)
   - Congenital adrenal hyperplasia
   - Some patients on cytotoxic drugs

What to give

- Major surgery: 200 mg/70 kg/day hydrocortisone phosphate
- Minor surgery: 100 mg/70 kg/day hydrocortisone phosphate

Reducing both 25%/day until normal oral steroids are resumed

Equivalent steroid doses (oral and intravenous)

	Duration of action (hrs)	Equivalent dose (mg)
Hydrocortisone (cortisol)	8–12	20
Prednisone	12–36	5
Prednisolone	12–36	5
Cortisone	8–12	25
Betamethasone	36–72	0.75
Dexamethasone	36–72	0.75

ANAESTHESIA AND ANTICOAGULATION

Background

Warfarin sodium is the most commonly prescribed oral anticoagulant; it acts by inhibiting vitamin K-dependent coagulation factors. The therapeutic range is a PTR of 2–4 times normal. Warfarin sodium can be reversed by vitamin K (takes 12 hrs to work).

Calcium heparin activates antithrombin III. Its half life is dose dependent (2–5 hrs). The therapeutic range is an APTT of twice normal. It may cause platelet consumption and emboli. Calcium heparin can be reversed with protamine sulphate (1 mg/100 IU heparin).

ANAESTHESIA AND ANTICOAGULATION (cont.)

Management of patient on long-term anticoagulants

1. Elective surgery
   a) Stop warfarin 2–4 days pre-operatively.
   b) Convert to intravenous or subcutaneous heparin, depending upon the degree of anticoagulation required (monitor APTT).
   c) Re-establish warfarin therapy post-operatively.

2. Emergency surgery
   Therapeutic doses of warfarin can be reversed with 0.5–1 mg vitamin K iv, checking PTR after 6 hrs (subsequent anticoagulation with warfarin may be difficult).
   Warfarin overdose or warfarin-related haemorrhage can be reversed with 2.5–20 mg vitamin K, although this takes up to 6 hrs to work and will render the patient resistant to the effects of warfarin for 2–4 weeks. Fresh frozen plasma (FFP) or freeze-dried prothrombin concentrate can be used to replace inactive factors acutely, although it will need repeating according to the PTR.

3. Liver failure
   A combination of platelet dysfunction and inactive vitamin K dependent coagulation factors may co-exist. Treat with FFP, vitamin K and platelets.

4. Central neural blockade and anticoagulation
   a) Avoid if patient is therapeutically anticoagulated with warfarin or iv heparin. (Recent use of aspirin and other non-steroidal anti-inflammatory agents is not a contraindication to central neural blockade).
   b) Omit subcutaneous heparin prior to epidural insertion/removal or spinal block.

ENDOCARDITIS PROPHYLAXIS

This is required for patients with heart valve defects (mitral valve prolapse only requires prophylaxis if there is a murmur), septal defects, patent ductus, prosthetic heart valves and possibly endocardial pacing wires.

Surgery or Instrumentation

Upper respiratory tract	As for dental cases
Genitourinary	Sterile urine – as for special risk group
	Infected urine – also include cover for identified pathogen
Obstetrics and gynaecology/ gastrointestinal	Prosthetic valve and previous endocarditis only (as for 'special risk group' dental cases)

PROPHYLAXIS FOR DENTAL SURGERY

Is patient in a special risk group ?

1. Prosthetic valve
2. Penicillin allergy
3. Penicillin more than once in previous month
4. Previous endocarditis

Yes →

Is the patient in group 2 or 3?

No ↓   Yes ↓

No ↓ (from special risk group)

---

amoxycillin
1 g iv/im
just prior to surgery and
500 mg orally
6 hrs later

5–10 yrs:
half adult dose

under 5 yrs:
quarter adult dose

or

amoxycillin
3 g orally 4hrs
prior to surgery
and 3 g orally ASAP
post-operatively

5–10 yrs:
half adult dose

under 5 yrs:
quarter adult dose

---

amoxycillin
1 g iv/im just prior
to surgery
500 mg orally
6 hrs later
and
gentamicin
120 mg iv/im
just prior
to surgery

5–10 yrs:
half adult dose of
amoxycillin, and
gentamicin
2 mg/kg

under 5 yrs:
quarter adult dose
amoxycillin, and
gentamicin
2 mg/kg

---

vancomycin
1 g iv over 1 hr
prior to surgery
and
gentamicin
120 mg iv/im
just prior
to surgery

under 10 yrs:
vancomycin
20 mg/kg and
gentamicin
2 mg/kg

or

teicoplanin
400 mg iv and
gentamicin
120 mg iv just
prior to surgery

under 14 yrs:
teicoplanin
6 mg/kg, and
gentamicin
2 mg/kg

or

clindamycin
300 mg iv
over 10 mins just
prior to surgery
and
150 mg orally/iv
6 hrs later

RESUSCITATION GUIDELINES

In recent years organisations such as the European Resuscitation Council and the American Heart Association have produced guidelines in an attempt to improve the standard of cardiopulmonary resuscitation. These are reviewed at intervals and changes made when justified. The most recent are the 1992 European Resuscitation Council guidelines (BMJ 1993, 306:1589–1593).There are three algorithms: one each for ventricular fibrillation, asystole and electromechanical dissociation. The new features introduced since previous recommendations are:

1. Each algorithm contains a loop to describe the actions to be taken if an arrest is prolonged.

2. The only drugs recommended in the algorithms are adrenaline and atropine. Other groups of drugs may be considered but particular drugs or doses are not specified.

3. In the ventricular fibrillation algorithm emphasis is placed on the importance of rapidly repeated defibrillation.

4. In prolonged asystole or electromechanical dissociation high dose adrenaline (5 mg) is recommended.

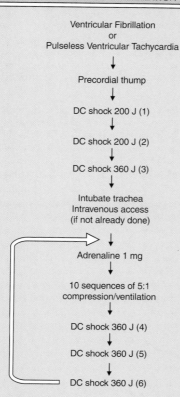

VENTRICULAR FIBRILLATION

Ventricular Fibrillation
or
Pulseless Ventricular Tachycardia

↓

Precordial thump

↓

DC shock 200 J (1)

↓

DC shock 200 J (2)

↓

DC shock 360 J (3)

↓

Intubate trachea
Intravenous access
(if not already done)

↓

Adrenaline 1 mg

↓

10 sequences of 5:1
compression/ventilation

↓

DC shock 360 J (4)

↓

DC shock 360 J (5)

↓

DC shock 360 J (6)

Notes
1. The interval between shocks 3 and 4 should not exceed 2 mins
2. Adrenaline should be given during each loop (i.e. every 2–3 mins)
3. Continue loops for as long as defibrillation is indicated
4. After 3 loops consider (i) an alkalizing agent
                           (ii) an anti-arrhythmic drug

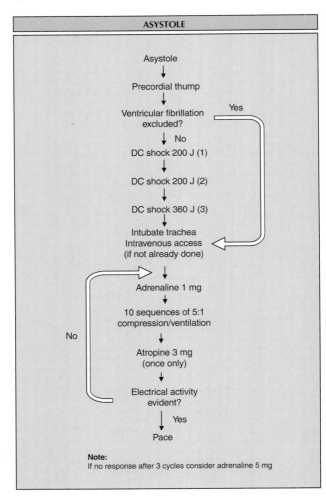

ASYSTOLE

Asystole
↓
Precordial thump
↓
Ventricular fibrillation
excluded?   Yes
↓ No
DC shock 200 J (1)
↓
DC shock 200 J (2)
↓
DC shock 360 J (3)
↓
Intubate trachea
Intravenous access
(if not already done)
↓
Adrenaline 1 mg
↓
10 sequences of 5:1
compression/ventilation
↓
Atropine 3 mg
(once only)
↓
Electrical activity
evident?
↓ Yes
Pace

No

Note:
If no response after 3 cycles consider adrenaline 5 mg

ELECTROMECHANICAL DISSOCIATION

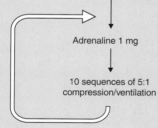

Electromechanical dissociation

↓

Consider and give specific treatment for:

Hypovolaemia
Tension pneumothorax
Cardiac tamponade
Pulmonary embolism
Drug overdose/intoxication
Hypothermia
Electrolyte imbalance

↓

Intubate trachea
Intravenous access
(if not already done)

↓

Adrenaline 1 mg

↓

10 sequences of 5:1
compression/ventilation

Note
Consider pressor agents, calcium,
alkalizing agents, adrenaline 5 mg

PAEDIATRIC RESUSCITATION

Basic Life Support		
	Infant	Child
	Clear the airway	Clear the airway
Breathing Initial Subsequent	2 breaths, 1 sec each 20 breaths/min	2 breaths, 1 sec each 15 breaths/min
Circulation ECM area Compressor Depth Rate C:V ratio	Lower third of sternum 2–3 fingers 2 cm 100/bpm 5:1 (ventilatory pause)	Lower third of sternum Heel of hand 3 cm 80–100/bpm 5:1 (ventilatory pause)

Asystole: most frequent cause of cardiac arrest in children, and usually results from respiratory arrest or hypovolaemia. Children with asystole are therefore often profoundly acidotic, early correction of which is considered important.

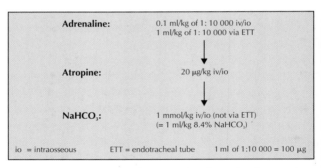

Adrenaline: 0.1 ml/kg of 1: 10 000 iv/io
1 ml/kg of 1: 10 000 via ETT

Atropine: 20 µg/kg iv/io

NaHCO₃: 1 mmol/kg iv/io (not via ETT)
(= 1 ml/kg 8.4% NaHCO₃)

io = intraosseous   ETT = endotracheal tube   1 ml of 1:10 000 = 100 µg

If no response occurs, continue high dose adrenaline, 100 µg/kg every three mins; outcome poor if no response occurs to second dose.

Ventricular fibrillation: uncommon in children but may be due to:

- hypothermia
- tricyclic overdose
- cardiac disease

Treat with asynchronous electrical defibrillation, as per algorithm opposite. Use paediatric paddles if < 10 kg (if unavailable, place apical adult paddle to left of sternum and the other on the back).

PAEDIATRIC RESUSCITATION (cont.)

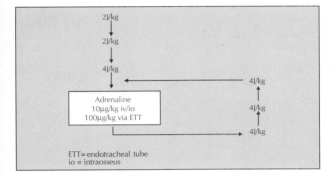

Electromechanical dissociation:

Always:	• Consider profound shock
	• Establish basic life support
	• Give 20 ml/kg crystalloid/colloid and adrenaline
Exclude:	• Pneumothorax
	• Tamponade
	• Pulmonary embolus
	• Hyperkalaemia/hypocalcaemia
Once excluded:	• Treat as asystole

RESUSCITATION OF THE NEWBORN

Principal problems

1. Failure to breathe

If heart rate < 80 bpm with intermittent breaths (no gasping) – intubate immediately, with two static inflations lasting 2–3 secs to peak pressure of 30 cmH$_2$O followed by IPPV, 30–40 breaths/min to peak airway pressure of 20 cmH$_2$O.

    a) Causes of apnoea:

- general anaesthetic
- pethidine – reverse with im naloxone; < 2 kg, 10 µg; > 2 kg, 20 µg
- hypocarbia
- severe acidosis/hypoxaemia
- hypoxic brain injury

RESUSCITATION OF THE NEWBORN (cont.)

b) Causes of persistent cyanosis:
- oesophageal/bronchial intubation
- pneumothorax
- diaphragmatic hernia
- severe hyaline membrane disease
- congenital heart disease

2. Severe bradycardia/asystole
- Most common cause is hypoxia
- commence external cardiac massage if heart rate < 40 bpm

Method: place thumb on midsternum and fingers along thoracic spine. Give 120–140 compressions/min, maintaining IPPV. Give adrenaline 10 µg/kg (= 0.1 ml/kg, 1:10 000) iv or 100 µg/kg (= 1 ml/kg, 1:10 000) via endotracheal tube.

3. Meconium aspiration

In presence of meconium-stained liquor, suck out mouth, oro-pharynx and nose prior to first breath. If the infant then:

a) coughs, cries and looks in good condition, take no further action.

b) looks in poor condition, DO NOT stimulate gasp, but visualise larynx and aspirate meconium from the trachea before commencing IPPV.

NEONATAL RESUSCITAIRE		
O₂ delivery system:	Self-inflating 250 ml bag/valve Premature and newborn size face masks	
Equipment:	Endotracheal tubes	< 0.75 kg 2.5 mm 1.75–3.5 kg 3.0 mm > 3.5 kg 3.5 mm
	Suction catheters 2 straight bladed laryngoscopes 5, 10 ml syringes Foil blanket Cannulae	
Drugs:	Naloxone (neonatal, 20 µg/ml) Adrenaline (1:10 000, 100 µg/ml)	

DIAGNOSIS OF BRAIN STEM DEATH

It is generally recognised that permanent functional death of the brain stem constitutes brain death. Collaborative efforts between various medical colleges have presented criteria for brain death, which are accepted as being sufficient to distinguish between those patients who retain enough functional capacity to have even a partial recovery and those in whom this possibility does not exist.

Pre-conditions for the testing of brain stem death

1. The patient MUST be deeply comatose
   (a) There should be no suspicion that the state is drug-induced.
   (b) Hypothermia should be excluded as the cause of coma.
   (c) Metabolic and endocrine disturbances which could be responsible for, or contribute to, coma should be excluded.
2. The patient MUST be ventilated because of the absence or inadequacy of spontaneous ventilation. Muscle relaxants and other drugs should be excluded as a cause of respiratory failure.
3. There should be NO DOUBT that the patient has suffered irremediable structural brain damage. A diagnosis of a disorder recognised to result in brain death should be fully established.

Diagnostic tests for the confirmation of brain death

All brain-stem reflexes must be absent; this is confirmed by fulfilment of the following criteria:

1. The pupils are fixed in diameter and do not respond to sharp changes in the intensity of incident light.
2. There is no corneal reflex.
3. The vestibulo-ocular reflexes are absent.
4. No motor responses within the cranial nerve distribution can be elicited by adequate stimulation of any somatic area.
5. There is no gag reflex or reflex response to bronchial stimulation by a suction catheter passed into the trachea.
6. No respiratory movements occur when the patient is disconnected from the mechanical ventilator for long enough to ensure that the P_aCO_2 is above the threshold for stimulation of respiration (normally 6.65 kPa, 50 mmHg).

Notes

1. Tests for brain-stem death should not normally be considered until at least 6 hrs after the onset of coma or, if cardiac arrest was the cause, 24 hrs after the circulation has been restored.

   The tests can be performed by neurologists or neurosurgeons and experienced clinicians in areas of intensive care, acute medicine or accident and emergency. The tests should be performed by two clinicians, namely, the consultant in charge of the case and one other doctor. In the absence of the consultant, his deputy may take responsibility providing he or she has been registered for ≥ 5 yrs and has adequate experience in this field.

DIAGNOSIS OF BRAIN STEM DEATH (cont.)

a) It is customary, but not essential, for the two doctors to repeat the tests in order to avoid observer error. Likewise there is no laid down time interval for the two sets of tests, which will depend upon the exact nature of the clinical problem.

b) Body temperature: Brain death tests should not be considered if the body temperature is < 35 °C.

c) Electroencephalography, cerebral angiography and cerebral blood flow measurements are not considered necessary for the diagnosis of brain stem death.

d) Vestibulo-ocular reflexes: Clear access to the tympanic membranes should be established by direct inspection. The reflexes are considered absent when no eye movement occurs during, or following, the slow injection of 20 ml ice cold water into each external auditory meatus in turn. (Local trauma may render this test impossible).

e) Apnoea: Respiratory movements must be demonstrated to be absent when the P_aCO_2 is above the threshold for stimulation of ventilation (Normally 6.65 kPa, 50 mmHg). The procedure taken depends upon whether blood gas analysis is available.

Blood gas analysis available:

- preoxygenate
- adjust ventilation to achieve P_aCO_2 of 5.3–6.0 kPa (40–45 mmHg)
- disconnect ventilator, preventing hypoxia by delivering O_2 6 l/min by passive flow into trachea
- look for respiratory effort while repeating blood gas analysis to ensure that P_aCO_2 threshold has been passed (P_aCO_2 will rise at 0.25–0.5 kPa/min)

Blood gas analysis not available:

- preoxygenate for 10 mins with 100% O_2, followed by 95% O_2/5% CO_2 for 5 mins
- disconnect patient from ventilator, delivering O_2 6 l/min by passive flow into trachea, and observe for 10 mins.

Patients with chronic CO_2 retention who normally exist on hypoxic drive require special attention.

MANAGEMENT OF ACUTE SEVERE ASTHMA
(adapted from Thorax, 1993; 43:Suppl S1–S24)

Features of acute severe asthma:
- Patient too wheezy to finish sentence in one breath
- Respiratory rate: > 25/min
- Heart rate: > 110/min
- Peak expiratory flow: < 50% predicted normal or recorded best

Features of life-threatening asthma:
- PEF < 33% predicted normal or recorded best
- Silent chest, cyanosis, feeble respiratory effort
- Bradycardia, hypotension
- Exhaustion, confusion, coma
- Blood gases: normal or rising P_aCO_2, falling P_aO_2, acidosis

Immediate management
1. O_2 – highest flow and concentration available.
2. Nebulised β_2 agonist: 5 mg salbutamol (children 0.15 mg/kg), or 10 mg terbutaline (repeated up to every 15 mins).
3. High dose steroid – hydrocortisone 200 mg iv 6 hrly.
4. Measure blood gases and exclude pneumothorax on chest X-ray.
5. In event of any life-threatening features, use:
   a) Nebulised ipratropium 0.5 mg 6 hrly.
   b) Aminophylline or β_2 agonist infusion:
      Aminophylline 5 mg/kg bolus slowly, followed by 0.5 mg/kg/hr (omit loading dose if patient on oral theophylline); therapeutic levels 55–110 µmol/l.
      Salbutamol 3–4 µg/kg bolus slowly, followed by 5–50 µg/min (until bronchospasm is broken or heart rate < 160 min).
6. Monitor S_aO_2 continuously and PEF, blood gases and serum K^+ intermittently.
7. Avoid sedation, antibiotics, percussive physiotherapy.

Intensive care
Patients with life-threatening asthma are best nursed in an intensive care environment with continuous ECG and S_aO_2 monitoring. Indications for ventilation include:
- Exhaustion, depressed conscious level
- Falling respiratory rate
- Rising P_aCO_2

Ventilation
Notoriously difficult, guidelines include:
1. The employment of full sedation and paralysis (avoiding histamine-releasing drugs).

MANAGEMENT OF ACUTE SEVERE ASTHMA (cont.)

2. Minimisation of airway pressures and gas trapping
   - small tidal volumes
   - long inspiratory and expiratory times → low respiratory rate
   - accept rising P_aCO_2.
   - manual chest compression to aid expiration may be life saving

3. Negative pressure ventilation, e.g. with the Cuirass Oscillator, may lessen the need for IPPV and aid weaning.

4. If unresponsive consider:

   a) Volatile agents – isoflurane, diethyl ether (beware of using halothane in view of hypercapnia and catecholeamines)

   b) Ketamine

   c) Inhaled local anaesthetics

   d) $MgSO_4$ iv

MANAGEMENT OF DIABETIC KETOACIDOSIS

Metabolic derangements include:
- Dehydration (up to 100 ml/kg)
- Electrolyte depletion (Na^+ 8 mmol/kg, K^+ 4 mmol/kg)
- Hyperglycaemia/hyperosmolality
- Metabolic acidosis with compensating respiratory alkalosis

Management:
Should take place in intensive care environment

1. Fluid and electrolytes

   a) Monitor urine output, core: peripheral temp gradient ± CVP.

   b) Give 0.9% NaCl   2 l in first hr
                          1 l in second hr
                          0.5 l/hr thereafter until well perfused

       i) If plasma Na^+ concentration is > 155 mmol/l on admission and one hr afterwards replace 0.9% NaCl with 0.45% solution after 3 l of 0.9% NaCl has been given.

       ii) Replace saline with 5–10% dextrose when blood sugar ≤ 10 mmol/l.

       iii) Give potassium according to following regimen:

Plasma K^+ (mmol/l)	KCl (mmol/l)
> 5	0
4–5	13
3–4	26
< 3	39

MANAGEMENT OF DIABETIC KETOACIDOSIS (cont.)

2. Insulin requirements

   Give 20 units of soluble insulin intravenously stat followed by 5–10 units/hr until blood sugar is approximately 10 mmol/l, then reduce according to the sliding scale to maintain blood sugar at 7–10 mmol/l.

3. Correction of acidosis
   - Only correct if pH < 7.1
   - Give 50 ml 8.4% $NaHCO_3$ with 13 mmol KCl over 30 mins
   - Check pH after 10 mins and repeat until pH ≥ 7.1

4. General management
   - Pass nasogastric tube (gastric dilatation common)
   - Give broad spectrum antibiotics
   - Take blood for FBC, U+Es, blood sugar, blood cultures
   - Catheterize, analyse urine for ketones, microscopy, culture and sensitivity
   - Chest X-ray
   - Continuous ECG (monitor T waves in particular) and S_aO_2
   - Repeat laboratory blood sugar and U+Es after one hour
   - Consider prophylaxis against DVT

5. Anaesthetic considerations
   - Rapid sequence induction (beware suxamethonium and hyperkalaemia)
   - Ventilate, continuing hyperventilation as respiratory compensation for metabolic acidosis
   - Monitor blood gases and blood sugar every 15 mins
   - Consider post-operative ventilation and admit to ICU

CHECKLIST FOR ANAESTHETIC MACHINE
(slightly modified from Association of Anaesthetists, 1990)

1. **Oxygen analyser/power**
   a) Position O_2 analyser on the common gas outlet and check its calibration.
   b) Turn on anaesthetic machine power supply; check monitor function and battery back-up, if fitted.

2. **Medical gas supplies**
   Start check with machine disconnected from pipeline supplies.
   a) Open all flowmeter controls.
   b) Turn on reserve O_2 cylinder, check contents gauge, check O_2 flowing in correct flowmeter. Repeat test on second cylinder, if fitted.
   c) Check O_2 flow valve, adjust over full range of flowmeter and set at a flow of approximately 5 l/min.
   d) Ensure that the O_2 analyser approaches 100%.
   e) Turn on reserve N_2O cylinder, check contents gauge and flowmeter. Repeat test on second cylinder, if fitted. Check flowmeter functions over the whole range and set at 5 l/min.
   f) Turn off O_2 cylinder(s), empty O_2 by operating the oxygen flush. Cylinder gauge should return to zero and the O_2 failure protection device function.
   g) Connect O_2 pipeline. Check pressure gauge reads 400 kPa, perform tug test to ensure probe is properly located.
   h) Turn off N_2O cylinder(s), connect pipeline, check pressure reading.
   i) Turn off all flowmeter valves.
   j) Operate emergency O_2 flush valve and check that there is no significant decrease in pipeline supply pressure. Confirm that the O_2 analyzer approaches 100%.

3. **Vaporizers**
   a) Check that the vaporizers are properly fitted and that the locking mechanism is engaged.
   b) Check that the vaporizers are filled and that the filling port is tightly closed.
   c) Set the O_2 flow rate at 6 l/min and temporarily occlude the common gas outlet. There should be no leak from the vaporizer fitments and flow meter bobbins should drop.
   d) Repeat test with vaporizer 'on'.

4. **Breathing systems**
   a) Inspect configuration of breathing and scavenging systems and check for leaks.
   b) Check valves can be fully opened and closed.

CHECKLIST FOR ANAESTHETIC MACHINE (cont.)

5. **Ventilator**
   a) Check that the ventilator controls are working.
   b) Occlude the ventilator port and check that the pressure relief valve functions correctly.
   c) Check that the disconnect alarm is present and operational. Ensure that there is an alternative means of ventilating the patient if the ventilator fails.
6. **Suction equipment**
   a) Ensure that suction equipment generates 'negative pressure' at the tip of the sucker.
7. **Ancillary equipment**
   a) Check the availability of functioning laryngoscopes, selection of tubes, catheter mount and suxamethonium.

PAEDIATRIC ENDOTRACHEAL TUBE SIZES			
Age/weight	Internal diameter (mm) (oral/nasal)	Length (cm)	
		oral	nasal
< 1.5 kg	2.5	10.5	13.0
1.5–3.5 kg	3.0	10.5	13.0
Term	3.5	11.0	14.0
3–12 mths	4.0	12.0	14.5
12–24 mths	4.5	13.5	15.0
> 24 mths	Age/4 + 4.5	Age/2 + 12	Age/2 + 15

N.B. These tables are guidelines only; a range of endotracheal tubes of varying length and diameter should always be available

MAPLESON'S CLASSIFICATION OF BREATHING SYSTEMS

		FGF to avoid CO_2 accumulation		Comments
		SV	IPPV	
A		Alveolar ventilation (60–70 ml/kg). Suitable for children > 25 kg (but requires 1–1.5 × minute ventilation due to lack of expiratory pause)	2 × minute ventilation	Magill; good but cumbersome for SV, poor for IPPV
Co-axial A (Lack)		Alveolar ventilation		Less cumbersome than Magill and has better scavenging potential. Modifications of original (↑ diameter, length) have improved performance.
B		2–2.5 × minute ventilation for both spontaneous and controlled ventilation		Often used for resuscitation, patient transfer and 'bagging', but high gas flows are required to prevent CO_2 accumulation.

MAPLESON'S CLASSIFICATION OF BREATHING SYSTEMS (cont.)

		FGF to avoid CO_2 accumulation		Comments
		SV	IPPV	
C		2–2.5 × minute ventilation for both spontaneous and controlled ventilation		As for Mapleson B
	Waters' cannister	Introduction of soda lime cannister renders circuit more efficient for SV and IPPV		Many disadvantages: cumbersome; variable dead space; potential airway exposure to soda lime

MAPLESON'S CLASSIFICATION OF BREATHING SYSTEMS (cont.)

	FGF to avoid CO₂ accumulation		Comments
	SV	IPPV	
D		Published recommendations vary from 70–300 ml/kg	Combination of minute volume and FGF determine $PaCO_2$, e.g, normocapnia achieved with FGF 70 ml/kg and ventilation of 150 ml/kg	D,E and F all T-pieces with identical performance. Bain particularly useful when access to airway is limited; also allows scavenging of expired gases. Accidental disconnection of the inner tube from its connector at the anaesthetic machine results in dangerous increase in deadspace. Bain not recommended for children <25 kg.
Co-axial D (Bain)		Suitable for children < 25 kg. Various recommendations for FGF a) 2.5 – 3 x MV b) 3 x (1000 +100 ml/kg) c) 15 x respiratory rate x wt	a) mechanical thumb: FGF = 2.5 – 3 x MV b) Flow generator: 1000 + 100 ml/kg if ventilation ≥ 1.5 x FGF	
E		Volume of expiratory limb ≥ 0.75 – 1.0 V$_T$		
F				The Jackson Rees modification (F) of the original Ayre's T-piece added an expiratory limb and open ended 500 ml reservoir bag to allow positive pressure ventilation. Its low resistance, dead space and weight account for its popularity in paediatric anaesthesia.

MEDICAL GAS CYLINDERS

Gas	Cylinder colour		Filling pressure		Pin code	Volume (largest standard Pin)
	Body	Neck	psi	kPa		
Oxygen	Black	White	1987	13700	2,5	680 (E)
Nitrous oxide	Blue	Blue	638	4400	3,5	1800 (E)
Entonox	Blue	Blue/white	1987	13700	a	5000(G)
Carbon dioxide	Grey	Grey	725	5000	1,6	1800 (E)
Cyclo-propane	Orange	Orange	65	500	3,6	180 (B)
Helium	Brown	Brown	1987	13700	4,6	300 (D)
Helium/oxygen	Black	Brown/white	1987	13700	2,4	N/A
Medical air	Grey	Black/white	1980	13500	1,5	640 (E)
Ethylene	Purple	Purple	1200	8268	1,3	—
5% Carbon dioxide/oxygen	Black	Grey/white	2014	13886	2,6	N/A

N/A = only available on special order

ASA CLASSIFICATION
(from NCEPOD report, 1991/2)

Class 1

The patient has no organic, physiological, biochemical or psychiatric disturbance. The pathological process for which the operation is to be performed is localized and does not entail a systemic disturbance, e.g. a fit patient with inguinal hernia, fibroid uterus in an otherwise healthy woman.

Class 2

Mild to moderate systemic disturbance or distress caused by the condition to be treated surgically or by other pathophysiological processes e.g., non- or only slightly limiting organic heart disease, mild diabetes, essential hypertension, anaemia. Others list extremes of age, obesity and chronic bronchitis.

Class 3

Severe systemic disease or disturbance from whatever cause, although the degree of disability may not be defined with finality, e.g. severely limiting organic heart disease, severe diabetes with vascular complications, moderate to severe pulmonary insufficiency, angina pectoris or healed myocardial infarction.

Class 4

Severe, life-threatening systemic disorders which are not always correctable by operation, e.g. patients with organic heart disease with signs of cardiac insufficiency, persistent angina, active myocarditis, advanced pulmonary, hepatic, renal or endocrine insufficiency.

Class 5

The moribund patient who has little chance of survival but is submitted to operation in desperation, e.g. ruptured aortic aneurysm with profound shock, major cerebral trauma with rapidly increasing intracranial pressure, massive pulmonary embolus. Most of these patients require operation as a resuscitative measure with little or no anaesthesia.

CEPOD CLASSIFICATION OF OPERATIONS

CEPOD 1   Immediate
Resuscitation simultaneous with surgical treatment, e.g. ruptured aneurysm. Operation usually within 1 hr.

CEPOD 2   Urgent
Operation as soon as possible after resuscitation, e.g. intestinal obstruction which requires correction of dehydration.

CEPOD 3   Scheduled
Early operation but not immediately life saving, e.g. cancer surgery.

CEPOD 4   Elective
Operation at a time to suit patient and surgeon, e.g. elective cholecystectomy.

ACKNOWLEDGEMENTS

Page 6. Acid-base diagram. Published by permission from **Anaesthesia** by WS Nimmo and G Smith (Volume 1), Blackwell Scientific Publications Limited, Oxford, UK.

Pages 8–9. Gaseous composition of respiratory gases and Gaseous composition of blood. Adapted from **Clinical and Resuscitative Data** by RPH Dunnill and MP Colvin (Third Edition) with permission from Blackwell Scientific Publications Limited, Oxford, UK.

Pages 15–16. Surface area nomograms. Adapted from **Documenta Geigy**, 1970 (Seventh Edition) with permission from Ciba Geigy Limited, Basel, Switzerland.

Page 20. Distribution of dermatomes. Adapted from **Clinical Anatomy for Medical Students** by Richard S Snell (Third Edition) with permission from Little, Brown and Company, Boston, USA.

Page 33. Infusion nomogram. Reproduced by permission from Dr GW Burton, Humphrey Davy Department of Anaesthesia, Bristol Royal Infirmary, Bristol, UK.

Pages 84–86. Figures adapted from **Anaesthesia** by WS Nimmo and G Smith (Volume 1) with permission from Blackwell Scientific Publications Limited, Oxford, UK.